KIDS & BOOZE

KIDS

& *What You Must Know to Help Them*

BOOZE

WILBUR CROSS

©1979

 A Sunrise Book
E. P. DUTTON · NEW YORK

Library of Congress Cataloging in Publication Data | Cross, Wilbur | Kids
& booze. | "A Sunrise Book." | Bibliography: p. 166 | Includes index. |
1. Alcohol and youth—United States. I. Title. HV4135.C76 1979 362.7'8'292
78-21105 | ISBN: 0-87690-355-3 (cloth) | 0-87690-314-6 (paper) |
Published simultaneously in Canada by Clarke, Irwin & Company Limited,
Toronto and Vancouver | Designed by Barbara Huntley | 10 9 8 7 6
5 4 3 2 1 | First Edition |

Contents

71883

Acknowledgments

Starting with the obvious, I am indebted in varying degrees to all of the people, institutions, and groups mentioned in this book. Many individuals cannot be thanked in print for their information, help, and encouragement because they prefer to remain anonymous.

Yet, at the risk of slighting some who contributed data, ideas, and dialogues during some three years of research, I particularly thank the following for their help and for the information, background materials, and sources they supplied: Rosemary Carmichael, Coordinator, Alcohol and Drug Program, District Ten, Bronx, New York; Lena DiCicco, Director, CASPAR program, Somerville, Massachusetts; Gary E. Fair, alcohol and drug consultant, Sedgwick, Kansas; Madonna C. Fullerton, Director of Alcohol Education at the University of Maine; Elva Herzog, Juvenile Section Psychologist, Piscataway, New Jersey; Timothy C. Hoover, Director of Youth Services, Pasadena (California) Council on Alcoholism; Nancy Howard, Co-Director of the Family Training Center, Columbia, Missouri; David J. Huberty, Coordinator of Detoxification at the Central Minnesota Health Center; Richard F. McLaughlin, Narcotic Coordinator, Board of Education of the City of New York; Eddie McNees, Outreach Coordinator, Mid-Cumberland Council on Alcohol and Drugs, Nashville, Tennessee; Gail G. Milgram, Director of Education, Center of Alcohol Studies at Rutgers University; Gary R. Olsen, Coordinator, Whitemarsh Youth Program, Pennsylvania; Terry J. Royer, health education consultant, Riverside, California; Don Samuels, Coordinator, PRIDE Program, Dade County, Florida; Marilyn Fusco Schlesinger, Coordinator of Youth Education and Counselling, Niagara County (New York) Council on Alcoholism; Alexandra Southerby, Southerby Associates, Long Beach, California; Richard Spoonster, Director, Alcohol Education Project of the PTA; Julie Stull of the National Clearinghouse for Alcohol Information; John F. Vickers, Youth Coordinator, Teen Alternatives Program (TAP) of Antelope Valley, California; Brian Windsor, Assistant Director, Alcohol Abuse Prevention, Boys' Clubs of America; Dolores F. Wright of the Division of General Welfare of the United Methodist Church; and John K. Zachariah, Counselor, The Center for Youth Services, Rochester, New York.

They, and the dozens of others who contributed, are the real "authors" of this book.

—Wilbur Cross

Introduction

You are reading this book because a son or daughter or another young person you care about has a drinking problem or appears to be headed for trouble. Perhaps you are also troubled because drinking among the young seems to be on the increase in your community and you have seen evidence that the situation is getting out of control.

Whatever the reason for your concern, you can be certain that this book will help you to focus more closely on the nature of the problem and determine what steps to take to correct it. I make no claim that I will present a neat, workable formula, or even that the book will answer most of your questions. But I will say that I have been closely, intimately involved with a wide range of drinking problems, that I have talked with hundreds upon hundreds of people who are similarly involved, and that this book reflects the thinking and attitudes and strivings of a great many young people whose lives have been changed because of their own firsthand acquaintance with booze. You cannot begin to solve any serious problem until you have a fundamental understanding of what the problem is all about, where it originated, and how it is affecting your life.

This book will not expound medical, psychological, and social theories. You can find many books on such theories in your public library.

This book will not expose you to scare stories and horror tales. Such sensational tidbits can easily be found in newspapers, magazines, and on radio and television.

This book will not rattle off statistics, despite the proliferation of facts and figures in governmental, professional, and technical journals—as well as in the public press.

Theories and formulas will not help you. Scare stories will not motivate problem drinkers to abstain. As for statistics, you are not concerned about 6.8 million people or 17.2 percent of all students in junior high schools in the Northeast, or one out of every seven females in the average community. The only statistic that has significance is one: *you.*

How does this subject affect *your* life, and what can *you* do about it?

That is what this book is all about.

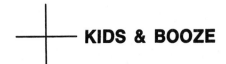 **KIDS & BOOZE**

1 What can be done to help the teenage problem drinker?

Kids and booze.

The idea is jolting, its implications disturbing. Think of a "kid"—an eighteen-year-old, a younger teenager, perhaps a child of nine or ten. Add "booze"—a highball, a shot of raw liquor, a little wine or beer—in quantities large enough to create problems for the persons drinking, and eventually for others with whom they are associated. Young people of various ages do drink, and do get into situations that range from mildly disconcerting to harshly disruptive—and in some cases hard to believe.

In this book real situations (not fictitious events although the names and locations may be disguised) are presented as a means of examining common problems and focusing on significant relationships that can help parents gain perspective and work toward realistic solutions. If a situation now seems *hopeless,* bear in mind that some of the most desperate drinking problems imaginable have been resolved, and some of the most incorrigible young alcoholics have been restored to normal, or near-normal, living.

Case #1. Dwight R. had been drinking since the age of ten, and heavily by the age of thirteen, when his parents were divorced and his father disappeared from his life. Since his mother was unable to exert any control over him, the youth was in frequent trouble with the law following drunken escapades. After a number of failures, a boys' club established rapport with Dwight and provided the guidance and support he needed. Today, in his mid-twenties, Dwight is an abstainer and a part-time counselor for the boys' club.

Case #2. Janice K. came from a fine home in a well-established community, living with her father, mother, sister, and brother. During high school years she drank nothing more than a little wine, an occasional beer. Yet by the time she was halfway through sophomore year at college she had acquired a reputation as the biggest party girl in the dormitory, frequently soused, and an easy target for males on the prowl. Her family might have remained unaware of her problem had they not received a notice from the dean's office announcing Janice's suspension for a month. When they drove in great distress to the college to pick her up, their daughter seemed to be a completely different person. Physically, she was a mess—haggard, bleary-eyed, and bloated. Mentally, she seemed unable to concentrate on anything, was exceedingly restless, and was constantly making up stories about people who were against her and telling lies about her. Suspension accomplished nothing. The family's ordeal continued for more than a year, with Janice drinking to greater and greater excess, unable to go back to college, hold a job, or even help out around the house. Finally, with the help of Alcoholics Anonymous and the guidance of an alcoholism counselor, Janice has managed to stay completely sober and is back in college, living a normal campus and social life.

Case #3. A suburban community near Boston was experiencing rough problems with the teenage population. Parents, having apparently overcome the crises of the pill-popping era, were hoping they could finally sit back and relax when they began realizing they were facing even greater threats from booze. High school students were bringing bottles of liquor to parties; school playing fields were littered with beer cans; youngsters in the seventh and eighth grades were passing out at picnics or arriving home staggering drunk. Disciplinary tactics, including curfews and off-limits zones, seemed to accomplish little more than to shift the drinking activities from one trouble zone to another. Through a coordinated effort on the part of parents, the school, the police, community agencies, alcoholism counselors, and others, the problems were resolved and a continuing alcohol education program was established.

You will encounter other such examples throughout this book. You will not find all the answers—no book could promise that—but you will discover that in a good percentage of cases of alcohol abuse by young people, there are sound reasons to hope for favorable responses to treatment.

What is the first step to take if your son or daughter has a drinking problem?

An experienced counselor with the New York City school system, Dick McLaughlin, makes a point you should keep in mind: Without wasting too much time determining who gets through to any particular youth, parents have to remember that *they* have the primary responsibility. If you have reason to believe that your child is having problems because of drinking, you may be tempted to say nothing and avoid making an issue of the subject for fear that you may arouse his curiosity and lead him to experiment with alcohol in a way that he might not have if left alone.

"This reasoning is dangerous. No matter how uncomfortable you may think a confrontation is going to be, the most sensible approach is for you to have a talk with your child immediately. It may be that you have been a very easygoing parent in the past, and have not talked seriously with your children about problems they are running into in the normal course of growing up. Thus, facing a crisis-motivated talk looms as a tough assignment. That is all the more reason for you to face up to the task. If you are going to deal with problems like alcohol abuse, you must function fully as a parent."

What if the confrontation explodes and your discussion is a complete bust? Don't panic. It frequently happens. Public school administrators, family consultation services, and other agencies mentioned in this book are among the resources that can help parents find a counselor who has had experience in dealing with young people who have become involved with drinking and drugs.

Can a counselor establish a sound working relationship?

It may seem ironic to you that a counselor, a complete stranger when he or she first enters the picture, might well be able to succeed where parents have failed. Yet we are familiar with this kind of developing relationship in the matter of doctors and psychiatrists and other professionals. So why not in the field of alcoholism and problem drinking?

As in any other career, there are plenty of individuals who are well qualified and effective, a few who are really outstanding, and a not surprising percentage who would have been better off going into some other calling.

"I cannot stress enough to any individual," says the director of youth services of the Pasadena (California) Council on

Alcoholism, Tim Hoover, "that if you have the slightest thought that someone you love or care about might have a drinking problem, *get to the professionals.*

"Find out what it is that you are up against and what positive actions you can take in order to help that person to reach help."

Despite his plea, which is echoed by many others who are knowledgable about problem drinking, there is one very common barrier across the land: *parental reluctance to seek such help.*

2 | How do you know if your child is a problem drinker?

Parents can go off half-cocked. They read scare headlines about the rise in drinking by teenagers. A seventeen-year-old daughter comes home looking glassy-eyed. An eighteen-year-old son passes out at a party and has to be carried home. Children, it seems, are slugging down uncommon amounts of beer these days and (even more disturbing) bottles of cheap wine. Parents are understandably disturbed when they hear this is going on behind their backs in the school yard, on campuses, or even in their own neighborhood.

If it is any comfort to you, a report published by the Rutgers Center of Alcohol Studies says that college students are neither drinking any more these days nor getting into any more alcohol-related trouble than they were a decade ago, or twenty-five years ago. "The proportions of students who are heavy drinkers or abstainers," said Dr. Ruth C. Engs of Indiana University, who conducted a nationwide survey on the subject, "appear to be about the same as the proportions in samples studied in the past."

Sadly, however, drinking *is* a problem in many cases. Usually the drinking has been going on for many months, perhaps years, without parents being any wiser until certain suspicious clues have come to light. How do you tell for certain whether you really need professional help or simply an old-fashioned face-to-face encounter to put the parental brakes on conduct that is getting out of hand?

Publications available from the government and from national organizations* frequently print checklists that are useful

* See the Appendix for details on publications and pertinent organizations.

in evalauting the situation. Here is a selection of questions compiled from a number of helpful lists and adapted specifically to the needs of parents:

1. Does your son or daughter show marked changes in regular habits and activities?

2. Has there been any trouble at school or with the police because of alcohol abuse, especially in situations that cannot be explained because of an inspiring sports victory or other local celebration?

3. Has much school time been lost for reasons that are not easily accountable?

4. Are grades steadily slipping, important exams being missed, or papers not prepared?

5. Have some regular friends been ditched or ignored in favor of others who seem inclined to drink or hang around?

6. Does your teenager evidence memory blanks about things that happened at a party or after drinking?

7. Are financial problems starting to surface?

8. Does your son or daughter show reluctance to discuss alcohol or talk about problems?

9. Have you been hearing any stories or rumors about how much your child is partying, or drinking, or goofing off?

10. Is there any evidence that he or she may be drinking alone, or sneaking drinks before going out?

11. Does your own liquor supply seem to be going down much faster than normal?

12. Is there any history of alcoholism in your immediate family, especially among relatives who are close to your children?

13. Conversely, is there parental pressure (because of religious, personal, or other reasons) to prohibit the use of alcoholic beverages of any kind?

14. Are there any severe or unusual pressures and stresses affecting family members at this time?

A "yes" answer to several of the questions does not prove that a drinking problem exists, but it does provide warning signals for you to consider.

If you are able to communicate reasonably well with your

teenager, ask him to answer—or at least consider in his own mind—the following questions:

1. Is my drinking pattern affecting my reputation at school or in the community—what my peers, teachers, and others are saying about me?

2. Do I drink to escape from pressures—studies, money, responsibilities, or other demands?

3. Do I drink to hide shyness or lack of self-confidence?

4. Do I need a drink before I go out to a social event?

5. When I go out on a date, does it seem to help to have a drink first, to overcome shyness or nervousness?

6. Do I get along with other kids better when beer, wine, or liquor is available and I can loosen up?

7. Do my friends generally drink less than I do?

8. Does it annoy or upset me when someone tells me I've had enough or too much to drink?

9. Do I feel guilty after drinking, or have a sense of great uneasiness the day after a party?

10. After drinking, are there things I cannot remember—a real memory block?

If you or your teenager honestly must answer "yes" to two or more of the questions on this list, you should consider that there is a problem that calls for corrective measures. No matter how many "yes" answers result, keep the situation in perspective. A young person (or an adult) could be reacting in a disturbing way to all of these questions, yet be far from becoming an alcoholic.

Is professional help necessary?

"Parents should act quickly and positively when there are clear indications that a son or daughter is having problems with alcohol," says Jack Drumwright, M.D., who serves as a physician and alcohol counselor at Continental Oil Company, "but they should not panic and they should never consider it a disciplinary matter. Criticism and condemnation have no place here—no more so than if an adolescent were getting poor marks in school because of a previously undetected hearing deficiency. Help the youth in any way you can and show that you *care*—but get professional help right away."

Some parents immediately express reservations about encouraging their children to join alcohol programs. Why? The problem has been put into focus by Marilyn Fusco Schlesinger, coordinator of youth education and counseling for the Niagara County (New York) Council on Alcoholism.

In dealing with alcoholic and alcohol-abusing adolescents, as well as with youths who are experiencing problems related to living with alcoholic parents, she has discovered that some are reluctant to inform their parents that they are being counseled because of a strong fear of being reprimanded. "It amazes me that a parent who does not have to think twice about sending a child to a medical doctor for physical care completely overlooks similar help for the child's emotional discomfort," says Schlesinger. "Many parents feel that emotional pain in youngsters will pass and is nothing to be alarmed about—that adolescence is a time of few pressures and little stress. Yet what might not be considered stressful to an adult may be a major catastrophe to a youth. Parents need to look at problems from their child's perspective and not their own.

"The first reason why some parents are reluctant to use counsel concerns the very idea of being a parent and the emotional investment made in parenthood. Most parents hope that they have raised a normal, if not 'perfect' human being. Could it thus be that they feel threatened by a counselor, who will conclude that their child is far from perfect and the problem is a direct result of poor parenting?"

If you are trying to resolve problems but feel threatened in this way, there is no need to overreact. "Most counselors," Schlesinger reassures us, "are not in the business of exposing parents as evil forces in a youth's life. They are instead working to improve communications between parents and children. Much of counseling involves listening, as well as educating people about new ways of coping, expressing themselves, and bettering their lives."

Invariably, counselors point out that communication can be established only when both young people and parents understand what it is like to be on the other side of the fence. It would seem that parents have a distinct advantage, since they were once teenagers but teenagers have never been adults. In most instances, however, counselors and alcohol coordinators constantly have to explain the differences in attitude and outlook.

Schlesinger says this procedure is "an examination of new methods of preventing problems from occurring in the future, not a process of finding fault with whatever has already happened."

As she points out, *all* families have problems. People must seek help when they have a problem that is interfering with their lives, and which they cannot solve individually or with help from their loved ones. What is needed in the case of young people who are experiencing alcohol-related problems is an atmosphere in which they can vent their feelings and discuss those problems openly. Parents must recognize that there will be times when they will not have the answers to their children's problems. At this point, counseling should be considered.

Why do young people drink?

There is no great mystery about why teenagers drink beer, wine, or hard liquor, and generally the problems are no more complex than the motivations. Many parents overreact, although some with serious problems often *under*react. We'll get into the problems later—the kids who drink as alcoholics, or the ones who become regular imbibers at the age of nine or ten. First, though, it is important to recognize what is normal drinking behavior. Gary E. Fair, a counselor in Sedgwick, Kansas, holds numerous rap sessions with teenagers. In these sessions, he focuses first on the reasons why the members of the group drink:

GARY: Why do you drink, each of you?

DEAN: To be sociable.

NORA: It relaxes you.

TONI: Because it feels good.

ALDEN: Sometimes, the taste. You have to learn to like the flavor of most drinks. Like drinking coffee. You're not born with a liking for it.

ROSE: Sometimes you play it straight and it's great. But then you want a variation. That's why kids drink sometimes.

GARY: When did you start drinking?

KEITH: At fifteen, fourteen, we used to go to the liquor store and buy stuff like candy-flavored brandy. The kid who lived up the block from us was our buyer. He was seventeen, but he looked eighteen and he'd buy it. We'd all have a party, with some stuff that was maybe 150 proof, and we used to buy all sorts of things like Gordons Vodka, and Seagrams Seven, and drink it straight.

GERRY: Right. We started drinking beer at about fifteen. Some people, adults I mean, got on our back, but it wasn't the same as if we'd been sneaking cocktails.

ELLIE: I started drinking when I was sixteen and my father said if he ever caught me drinking before I was twenty-one, he'd take away all my privileges. I'm obstinate, I admit it. So I sneaked drinks just to see how much I could get away with. Then somewhere I read a frightening article about alcoholics, which said that a high percentage of them came from families where drinking was forbidden. Like the Mormons—few of them drink, it said, but about one out of every two that do is a problem drinker. I guess because the feelings of guilt are all mixed in and activate some kind of bad reaction. So I quit cold and I never have anything except maybe a few sips of champagne at a wedding, when there's a toast.

You can logically blame curiosity as the urge that leads to the first taste, rather than an instinct to be naughty or deliberately disobedient. Generally, most kids dislike the taste of alcohol and, if left to their own preferences, would avoid the stuff as instinctively as if it were bitter medicine.

Among teenagers who drink, the reasons are generally quite normal, at least among those who are not suffering from any alcohol-related problems. A dozen eighteen-year-olds in Illinois who were getting ready for college discussed the subject. None of the members of this group is in trouble because of drinking, although several admitted that they had been drunk on occasion. Most felt that they could have become problem drinkers—or might in the future—if faced with problems that led them to the bottle as an escape, or if they developed some as-yet-unknown chemical imbalance that triggered an addiction.

What do young people drink?

LOU: Beer is most popular. It's easy to get. Convenient. You don't feel like you're a "drinker," I mean drinking for the sake of proving something to someone. I drink two or three cans, mostly at parties. Once in a while, more.

NOLA: I don't like beer except when it's real hot out and I'm thirsty. Mostly, of course, we have parties at night, that is, when beer is available and it's not hot. I'll get through one can at a party. That's all. I like wine much better, but only at meals because we have it at home on occasions.

JAN: I have a married sister and when I go over to her apartment she and her husband usually offer me a cocktail. I've been drinking cocktails or tall drinks for about two years. One, though, that's all. The most I ever had was two and I didn't like the feeling of being kind of out in space. My sister gets kind of silly when she drinks, but I don't think she has any problem. She's been drinking about seven or eight years and never has more than three drinks in an entire evening. I don't like beer. When I go to a school party, that is, with classmates, I drink Tab or Dr Pepper.

JIM: I got to like beer when I was on a construction job last summer. All the guys had beer for lunch. It was something new for me. I went along with them as though it had been a regular drink with me. But I started to get a beer belly. I really did. You read about that, but it's true. And I'm on a couple of varsity teams so I'm mostly in training during the school year. It'll probably be the same at college.

How do young people get started drinking?

"If you're a young man or woman in your teens," says a booklet prepared for young people by the Department of Health, Education and Welfare (HEW), "you know that teenagers do drink. No matter how you yourself feel about drinking, you're aware that some young people use alcoholic beverages."

This fact is accepted by the young, but it often surprises or even terrifies many adults, whose thinking is locked into the idea that the legal age for drinking in most states is twenty-one, and certainly no lower than eighteen or nineteen in others. It is hard for them to accept the fact that teenage drinking does occur quite commonly, and even more difficult to discuss the subject without becoming uptight.

HEW's evaluation of the situation is that a majority of teenagers in the country have "used" alcoholic beverages before getting out of high school—anything from a single drink to fairly regular weekend beer parties. But there are wide variations, depending upon such factors as community customs, religion, cultural background, educational programs, family habits, and the accessibility of beer, wine, or liquor. Your community may have as high a proportion as 80 percent, or as low as 20 percent, of young people who have "used" alcohol in some form.

At what age does drinking begin?

Most adults seem to picture a sixteen- or seventeen-year-old when thinking about that first drinking experience. Realistically, it occurs much earlier. If parents drink, or if wine is served on the family table, the age is almost certain to be at least thirteen, or more likely preteen.

According to Dr. Ross Fishman of the National Council on Alcoholism, children have learned about drinking by the time they reach the age of twelve. That does not necessarily mean that they have tasted liquor in any form, but rather that they have gathered impressions about what liquor is and what it does, or does not, do to a person. Just as children learn to understand a language before they are able to speak it, so they learn about beer, wine, and alcohol. And as with language, when they actually start using it they may do it poorly or well, positively or negatively, depending upon how effectively they have been educated.

The real facts about the age at which drinking begins often strike people in such a way that they react with disbelief.

"I was shocked to learn that we have youngsters—even eight years old, nine, or ten—who are drinkers. They leave home and go to school and somewhere along the way they get wine and sip it all day.

"And the parents are not even aware of this. How can this be?"

The shocked voice was that of an interviewer on a Pittsburgh radio station, questioning Ken Ramsey, director of the Gateway Rehabilitation Center in Pittsburgh, Pa., on teenage drinking problems. The interview was characteristic of radio and television broadcasts that are being aired with increasing frequency as the subject of alcohol use and abuse comes more and more out into the open.

Ramsey was asked what kinds of signs (other than the obvious ones) indicate that a young person has been drinking. He replied that a parent has to be close to a child to detect some of the more subtle indications, such as redness in the eyes or a spaced-out look. If a child is imbibing habitually, the giveaways may be changes in attitude about school and schoolwork, life at home, friends, or people in general, or an insistence on sharing or sipping drinks whenever adults are having beer, wine, or liquor.

Is drunken behavior a problem?

One of the vicious truths about heavy drinking is that although older people may take years to slide downhill from social drinking to alcoholic drinking, teenagers can reach that low point in as little as a year's time—especially if they are also taking other drugs.

There are two fundamental reasons why teenagers take up drinking, in the opinion of one counselor. The first is peer pressure by the young people they associate with. The other is what he calls the "indestructible concept"—the conviction that alcoholism will never happen to them and the feeling that the kids who are having fun and going to parties are the ones who drink a lot.

"Many of these kids don't view their drinking as a problem," said a therapist who works with the Fairfax, Virginia, Alcohol Safety Action Program (ASAP), "even though they have been arrested."

The subject was explored by one group of young people addressing themselves to the question, "Drunken Behavior—Is It Ever Acceptable?" Here is how two of them felt about it:

ALEX: If I'm drunk, should I be accepted, is that what you mean? Why not? Isn't it okay if I drink as much as I want to? It's my own affair.

ROSE: No, because your drunkenness isn't your own affair. It affects a lot of others—your family, friends, others. Even society. One guy told me at our last talk-out that 40 percent of all crimes were related to drinking.

ALEX: I'm talking about just being grossed, like at a party, and I'm wedged into a corner and not bothering anybody. Sure, we got to be responsible for our actions. And if we get corked we got a big headache the next day and serves us right. But you—you don't have my headache! I still think it's okay if you get drunk, get as plastered as you want to, at home. It's a place where you've got nobody watching you. You're not with a bunch of strangers.

ROSE: So your standard is that if you're with people you know, it doesn't matter? It all depends on who's watching you?

ALEX: At home, you're not degrading yourself. It's different if you are out at a bar. You have people seeing you and the next day you think back on what you were like in public. I've gotten drunk in front of friends and they don't go around feeling something's freaky. They've done the same thing. Everybody has a good time and they don't feel anything except that's what they're there for.

How do young people get booze?

Adults are often surprised that youngsters are able to obtain alcoholic beverages. Yet children well below drinking age are very knowledgable when it comes to locating sources of supply. Some seventh-graders were described as frequenters of supermarket parking lots, hanging around until some acquaintance came along who was old enough, and cooperative enough, to go in and purchase six-packs of beer. Parents more often than not never suspect that children this age could possibly obtain beer, wine, or liquor. And if a twelve- or thirteen-year-old is obtaining a supply, he will almost invariably set his parents' doubts at rest by assuring them, "No, I'm not fooling around with booze."

Young members of Alcoholics Anonymous talk openly about their introductions to booze and some of the ingenious or painstaking ways in which they managed to obtain beer, wine, or hard liquor when they were obviously way under age. Rick used to burrow under the fence of a nearby brewing company where he found bottles of beer that still contained enough dregs —though flat and warm—to get him high. Jan rode on her older brother's coattails until she found that there were plenty of males of legal drinking age who would buy her beer or whiskey if she expressed a desire to get loaded.

Bernice took on baby-sitting jobs for couples who had well-stocked bars. She never drank on the job, but filled flasks she had concealed in the knapsack she used to carry her school books. Caught in the act one evening when the flask leaked as she was going off the job, she came up with a tall tale that she had found it in a friend's car and was planning to turn it over to her parents so there would be no possibility of drunken driving.

Larry took a bolder approach. He patiently waited in the parking lot of a shopping center, near a liquor store. Eventually some customer would emerge from the store who would plunk his purchase in the front seat of a parked car, then dash back into a store for something he had forgotten. At the right moment, Larry would ride by on his bike, deftly transfer the package of liquor into his handlebar rack, and be off. "It was easy," he says, "all a matter of timing. Only one man ever saw me and shouted, and by then I was too far away."

Isn't alcohol too expensive for most youngsters to buy?

Adults believe this, but young people have a different system of economics:

ALAN: Booze is cheap, especially beer. And if you have several guys involved you can have a "kegger" and make everyone pay a couple of bucks.

FRED: Kids buy mostly for themselves or it's a chip-in. Especially, it's not out of line when you think what you pay for a chocolate frost or a cheeseburger. Just give up the frost—have a couple of beers. Some six-packs are cheaper than Coke.

PARENT: You're talking about beer. But how do you get wine or whiskey if you're underage or can't crib an I.D. card?

HOWARD: Easy. Every kid has a friend who is older, who went through the same hassle. So he says sure, why not, and takes your money and goes into the liquor store and gets whatever you want.

DANNY: You'll always find some dude who wants to make a couple of bucks, too, if you're really stuck. You give him payment for a bottle of wine and a crock of whiskey, plus about 20 percent "carrying charge." It's that simple.

Can teenage drinkers really be alcoholics?

Actions speak louder than words. These are typical comments from young people barely into their teens who described numerous experiences with drinking:

GREG: The first time I got wiped out I was twelve. My older brother was having a blast. He didn't want me around, but I snuck in and snatched a beer. One of the older guys gave me my second beer and what I didn't know was, he'd needled it with vodka. I got sick and puked all over and my mother was so pissed off she broke a broom over my head. I never felt a thing.

You'd think that experience would have ended my thirst for booze, but it didn't. There was some kind of mania—maybe suicidal—

that got me into other situations just like this one. The big kids thought it was a gasser to get me bombed. Finally I did too.

CARLOTTA: Wine did good things to me when I was in about ninth grade. We always had a bottle of red on the table and it gave me a warm glow inside. I really had good vibes. It lasted about a year and then it began making me nervous. I'd get twitchy if I didn't have a couple of glasses, if I was out somewhere away from home and there wasn't any wine. So I used to make sure I had a bottle stashed away or with me. If I went to a friend's overnight I'd take a bottle. At first it was just wine. Then rye or gin. I hated rye and gin, but after the first drink it didn't matter. The health angle I think of is that it creeps into your system without your knowing it, like maybe an infection spreads and you can't control it.

What makes young people drink too much?

"There is no simple answer," says Dick McLaughlin, the Brooklyn alcohol coordinator mentioned earlier. "About 90 percent of those who use alcohol have no real problems with it. The 10 percent that do persist in the illusion that they are in the normal group. So a major problem is the lack of insight into one's own condition."

At William McKinley Junior High School 259, which comes under his jurisdiction, Dick issues information sheets and educational bulletins that are jam-packed with facts, examples, suggestions, and quotes from reliable specialists in the field. Of special interest is his outline of nine major reasons why young people in junior high and high school become involved with alcohol. Somewhat condensed and edited, here is the sum and substance of what he has to say based on solid personal experience:

1. Curiosity. Young people like to experiment. They want to try something new and usually there are plenty of drinks and types of drinks they have never sampled.

2. Peer-Group Pressures. Everyone else is drinking, so why be a drag? That outlook encourages many a youth to drink beyond his capacity.

3. Escape from Everyday Problems. Alcohol offers a temporary escape from painful family relationships, the absence of love and affection.

Disappointments in boy-girl relationships often trigger an escape to alcohol.

Drinking seems to help in the adjustment to adolescent physiological changes—growing pains. How often do adolescents look at themselves in the mirror? If they don't like what they see there, they may seek some form of escape.

4. Mass-Media Saturation. Newspapers, magazines, radio, and television all glamorize drinking as a kind of status symbol. The ones who do the drinking tend to be virile men, gorgeous women, or famous personalities.

5. Availability. This includes not only the opportunities to obtain beer, wine, and liquor, but the accepted locations in which to consume it.

Are your children visiting these places?

6. Lack of Goals. As concerned adults, have we really helped our children to establish goals—that is, *attainable* goals?

Are we helping our young people to achieve these goals in high school? at college? in a career?

7. Rebellion. We see two extremes in the spectrum of discipline. The first is an excessive, tyrannical discipline that breaks down the communication system between parent and child and literally forces the child to seek comfort and understanding outside the home.

The other extreme is the lack of discipline, which leads youngsters to reject their parents because of a lack of respect for them.

We hear often about rebellion against parental authority, but we do not take into account the impact of the rebellion against parental *indifference.*

8. Questionable Morality of the Adult Culture. Have you ever noticed how many bars you walk past in a day? Have you ever been invited to a party where the host did not serve alcoholic beverages?

Alcoholism accounts for 60 percent of the admissions to mental hospitals, ranks second as a cause of suicide in the United States, contributes significantly to family discord and emotional disorders, and costs thousands of jobs and huge losses to our economy.

How many X- or R-rated movies have your children been

to lately—or do you know? Do you read the reviews before you send your youngsters off to the movies?

Do family members attend church services together? Is religion discussed at home?

9. Lack of Communication. How often do family members sit down and discuss their mutual problems? Do you talk wtih your children about where they have been and how they enjoyed themselves after being out at a party or with a date in the evening?

How often do you engage in person-to-person talks with your sons or daughters?

Do you really *listen* when your children are talking, to acquire some idea of the numerous problems they encounter in their daily lives?

What's wrong with drinking for pleasure?

The millions of adults who drink moderately without any problems have no doubts that beer, wine, and liquor can add considerably to the enjoyment of living. Why shouldn't young people who are of legal age and not constrained by religious or ethnic bans find this same enjoyment? Unless you are a teetotaler, this sounds like a reasonable argument. But very often professional counselors respond to other arguments that are considered to be equally relevant.

• Why involve a teenager in what might turn out to be a bad habit if he or she shows no natural inclination to drink?

• Is the young person *mature* enough, regardless of age?

• Aren't kids too inexperienced to start drinking, except under very controlled circumstances?

• Isn't it tough to get a young person to learn about alcohol and have a healthy respect for what it can do?

• Don't some of the emotional characteristics we associate with teenagers, such as excitability, enthusiasm, rebellion, changing moods, and lack of self-confidence, make it more risky for them to drink alcoholic beverages than for adults?

• Since a person's size and weight partially determine how much alcohol can be absorbed before inebriation takes over, aren't teenagers at a great disadvantage until they have attained full growth?

 • Isn't it true that although most adults are plagued with a few friends who try to push drinks on them, young people are likely to be subjected to a great deal more of this kind of pressure?

How should parents teach young people about drinking?

Parents have to be close enough to their kids to establish a good communications pipeline, even though drinking is an area of special sensitivity, involving a tendency to secretiveness and an astonishing lack of knowledge about booze and its effects.

When parents—usually unwittingly—dispense *mis*information to their children, they not only head them in the wrong direction but may very well weaken their rapport by undermining their credibility. Often parents are reluctant to discuss alcohol and alcoholism openly. Emotional conflicts flare up whenever and wherever the subject is discussed by people who are not knowledgable, and there remains a lingering belief that alcoholics are weak-willed and that alcoholism is not a disease but a disgrace.

Writing in a medical journal, Dr. Marvin A. Block, a member of the American Medical Association's committee on alcoholism, observed:

After addressing a class of university students on the subject of alcoholism and drugs, I was accosted by a young lady with a question I have been asked many times. "They teach us many things in school," she remarked, "but tell me, Doctor, why is it that they don't teach us how to meet life?"

That's a good question. But after all, teaching the young how to meet the problems of living is only partially a proper function of the school. Such instruction is to a far greater extent a parental responsibility. Specifically, when certain young people turn to drugs or become alcoholics, the school cannot justly be blamed for their tragedy; the fault may lie with parental neglect.

Are there good, as well as bad, reasons for drinking?

We get so uptight about the problems of drinking that we often ignore the reasons why alcoholic beverages have been developed and refined over hundred and hundreds of years: for pleasure and relaxation, as well as to enhance and add another dimension to dining. A group of high school students in the California wine-growing region, ages sixteen to eighteen and all of them in trouble because of alcohol abuse, were asked if there are good and bad reasons for drinking. Here are some of their responses:

JOSE: *Bad* because I got sick, sick, sick from drinking. *Good* because my father wouldn't have a job if there was no wine business.

LISA: I got in a mess of trouble because I got into beer, and that was okay until someone spiked it and I got hooked on hard stuff and started drinking it—but like beer. I messed up my life last year but now I don't drink anything except wine, and then when I'm having something to eat. My mother and father drink wine at meals. They enjoy it and they let me drink wine at the table anytime. But they never really knew how much misery I made for myself before.

SHARON: Isn't one of the major benefits of alcohol the way it is used for recipes? French chefs use wines and brandy in all kinds of dishes. They produce the best foods you can get at restaurants.

NEIL: I think the bad part is peer pressure. I wouldn't have drunk and got suspended if it hadn't been for guys who kept saying, "Are you Neil or Nellie? Have a slug. Or chug-a-lug." I was a year, two years younger so I thought it was smart to copy the seniors. I was a soph. But if you want a good scene, I say what about a good cold beer, maybe two, on a real hot day while you are at the ball park!

VINCENT: Or when you're on the ski slopes and it's about ten below zero or seems like, and you come into the lodge and have a hot buttered rum. Just one, not to get smashed. I only had one, one time at Squaw. But it could be a Black Russian. A nog. Just for that warm burner inside. Not to make you feel like your head's on backwards the next day.

GLORIA: We forgot. You have to have champagne at a wedding, or it isn't a real wedding.

NEIL: A lot of kids get stoned at weddings, on champagne.

GLORIA: Okay, it's good and it's bad at the same time. If you drink it right, it's good. If you slop it down like a pig, it's bad. You could say that for milk shakes. A friend of mine is a big, fat, sloppy mess. She drinks milk shakes like it would make anyone else throw up. I can't stand to watch her gulp shakes. You know, if each one had an ounce of liquor, she'd be bombed all the time.

Why do we need to know more about alcohol?

A special report to Congress by the Department of Health, Education and Welfare recently made this revelation, which has justifiably been described as "striking": Light drinkers or people who abstain were found to *know* a lot more about alcohol and the effects of alcohol than people who were heavy drinkers or problem drinkers. What that means is that if you *know* the pitfalls, you're going to avoid them. Unless you have some chemical imbalance that makes you really an alcoholic, you are going to be able to drink properly—and enjoy what you drink.

Do the experts say teenagers should or should not drink?

"On the controversial subject of liquor," says one counselor, "you find only one point that the experts all agree on: uncontrolled drinking leads to trouble and causes problems. Physicians, counselors, psychologists, educators, researchers— they all have different theories and often disagree with each other point-blank. So you alone have to weigh the factors and be the judge." As an example, here are some statements which seem simple and direct enough to reach an agreement on, but which are in fact highly controversial:

"The best rule is that teenagers should not be allowed to drink at all."

Pro: Using alcohol in any form is wrong. Banning it entirely is the best answer.

Con: Prohibition does not work for any age group, teenagers or adults. It has been demonstrated that many alcoholics come from families or communities where drinking is banned.

"Teenagers should be allowed to drink, so that they can learn to drink in moderation."

Pro: If parents permit drinking in the home, such as wine at dinner or an occasional cocktail that is properly mixed, they can educate their children properly so they will know how to handle drinks when they are outside the home.

Con: Permitting drinking is the same as encouraging it. Why suggest starting this bad habit any more than you would hand cigarettes to your children and encourage them to smoke?

"Teenagers cannot handle alcohol. Only by the age of twenty or twenty-one is a person mature enough to drink."

Pro: Adolescents use alcohol indiscriminately and unwisely. By the time they reach adulthood they have already established bad drinking habits that they cannot change.

Con: That's all wrong because young people are generally responsible and eager to do things the right way. No one advocates postponing a person's education until he has reached twenty or twenty-one on the assumption that he will "mislearn" the subjects of his school courses.

"Adolescence is actually too late to start learning to drink. The best way is to let young children have an occasional sip of wine or beer at home with their parents."

Pro: When youngsters first become acquainted with alcohol this way, they do not grow up with the misguided idea that it is mysterious or glamorous, but simply on a par with other beverages or foods, to be used moderately and properly.

Con: It sounds logical, but it doesn't work that way. Look at France, which has an enormous national drinking problem. There, young children are brought up having wine (and diluted with water at that!) at meals.

"The best way for parents to make sure that their children do not have drinking problems is for them to be teetotalers themselves, at least during the period when their children are growing up."

Pro: Young people tend to respect the wishes of their parents better if what the parents do is consistent with the policies they try to establish.

Con: Unfortunately, there are many, many cases of teenage alcoholics whose parents are teetotalers. They go to parties where everyone else is having beer, succumb to peer pressure to have just one, and then undergo feelings of guilt which eventually lead them to drinking as an escape.

4 | *How do parents' drinking habits influence their children?*

Some adults will admit that their own drinking habits are not always above reproach. Yet what really escapes their understanding is that children will imitate their elders in numerous ways, not excluding the intake of alcoholic beverages. It is thus disturbing to realize that the "knowledgable" and sophisticated adult is often considered to be that congenial neighbor who knows how to mix the perfect martini, serves beer in frosted mugs, buys liquor at discounts you didn't know were possible, and has a flair for serving exactly the right wines at the dinner table.

The Boys' Clubs of America (BCA) touched on this subject at a meeting in which adults and young people were brought together to air mutual concerns and learn about gaps in their attitudes and beliefs.

PARENT: I suppose you'd have to say one reason why young people drink is because they see their parents drinking. I can't very well drink cocktails every evening and then try to tell my son he'll go to hell if he follows suit.

FRED: True. If you, if parents label alcoholic beverages "acceptable," then kids do it, too.

PARENT: Look at it the other way around, though. It seems to me that when a parent labels it "*un*acceptable," maybe because he has religious convictions or thinks it's dangerous to the health, a lot of teenagers then get rebellious. In other words, they want to do what the parent does if he drinks, but they don't want to follow in his footsteps if he doesn't drink.

ALAN: No, I don't agree. I respect what you say, but this kind of rebellion you mention is some other kind of animal. If a parent does not drink, and has a reason for it besides just being stuffy, a kid will respect that viewpoint and maybe even adopt it himself—but later. He'll probably experiment a little with beer and wine, maybe liquor. But there's a chance he'll say the old man is right, why bother with all this stuff? It's when the parents make a big deal of not drinking or try to paint it like robbing a bank or streetwalking that they lose the kids out in left field.

PARENT: Is "peer pressure" a valid reason why teenagers—some teenagers—drink?

DANNY: Let me throw the question right back at you, Mrs. T. Is "peer pressure" a reason why some adults go to a party and get loaded when they had intended drinking gingerale? Sure, the answer is "yes." But for any age, not just those under twenty.

PARENT: True, but I think adolescents are more apt to be pressured than adults are. Perhaps I should say that the adults who are that easily pressured actually never did grow completely out of their teens.

DANNY: It's an escape, too. That's a good reason. Teenagers have a lot of things they're trying to escape from. Like stress.

PARENT: What makes you think teenagers have a corner on that market? or lack of confidence? or feelings of being rejected? or any other of the deficiencies that make older people start drinking too often and too much?

DANNY: Well, it *is* a reason.

"Of all these reasons why young people drink," says a report issued by BCA, "perhaps the most influential is that they see their parents do it. The fact that parents' practices strongly determine their children's drinking patterns has several implications to those of us in alcohol-abuse prevention. We must bear in mind that the two groups of children who run the highest risk of having alcohol-abuse problems are those with one or more alcoholic parents, and those whose parents are teetotalers."

Here are some ways in which young people evaluated the drinking habits of their own parents:

GRIFF: My father is all right. I'm probably the same way. He sits around the house and drinks Millers or Bud, mostly on Fridays and Saturdays. Then he'll get up, if he's in the living room, and go into the kitchen and watch Mom cooking and talk.

COLETTE: My father (he's thirty-nine) and mother go out to a lot of parties. They are very social, and he drinks but is okay, even if a little tipsy sometimes. They jazz around a bit after they come home and have fun.

RAY: I'd like to drink like my mother. She knows when to quit and she never drinks too much. She can hold it. That's the way I'd like to drink. I don't always. Usually she drinks at home. When I drink, I like to do it at home. I don't like to go out. It's more comfortable.

CHRIS: My folks are probably the most accomplished social drinkers in town. Every night, promptly at 5:30, the booze comes out and they party. Dancing at the club. Dancing here and there, running all over. I really love their life-style. They get squiffed enough so everyone's having a good time. Not squashed. They get home. They hit the sack and they're up the next morning going to work. And then at 5:30 the next day they're off again. Almost seven days a week. I don't know how they do it, but it's a great way to go.

Are the families of problem drinkers trouble-prone?

In families affected by drinking problems, one of the common denominators is a lack of action. Gary Fair, the counselor in Kansas, who has worked with alcohol education programs for some fifteen years, deplores the fact that people wait so long to take any steps when drinking problems develop. "The average family waits seven years," he explains. "Would you believe it—seven years from the time a drinking problem is first suspected before dealing with it. Then the members of the family go through all kinds of torment trying to solve the problems. It seems to be human nature that we do not fight the problems initially. We wait until they become acute.

"Now take the case of a father who hits the bottle. It becomes apparent but no one does anything, beyond the usual arguments. By the time steps are taken, the man may have lost his job, become ill, had auto wrecks. Finally the alcoholic father does become sober and on the way to recovery. But by then the wife has taken to drink, probably left home, and is in bad shape. The kids are in bad shape emotionally, as well as financially, so maybe they're starting to drink. It all becomes a lifetime problem and no way anyone can put it all back together again."

In his contacts with teenagers whose problems have been caused by a parent or other member of the family who is drinking heavily, Gary has noted that sometimes these young victims are really sicker than the alcoholics. "They crack under the strain," he says, "because they have to cope with the irate phone calls, the unpaid bills, the mess, the problems. Alcoholics will get rid of every bit of responsibility. That's the way their minds operate and you cannot rationalize. The sooner the family realizes this and seeks help, the sooner some of the problems can be resolved. It's the waiting, the delay, that compounds all of these problems."

A professional counselor can help to evaluate a young person who has problems that are largely alcohol-related. One such counselor is John K. Zachariah, who specializes in drug and alcohol abuse at the Center for Youth Services in Rochester, New York. In most of the cases of adolescent drinking that he has dealt with, the most significant overall characteristic is what he refers to as "locus of control"—a belief in the degree to which a person is responsible for his own reinforcements. Those with drinking problems tend to place responsibility on others who are more powerful than they are, or on forces they cannot control.

One young drinker attributed his inability to control his abuse of alcohol to his faulty personality: "I'm powerless over booze, drugs, cigarettes, pinball machines, and anything else that can be addictive."

Another was convinced that trying to change drinking behavior was a useless exercise for an alcoholic: "No matter what attitudes our parents take, or how they rap with us, or don't rap, we still got diabetes. Only in our case it's alcoholism. Everyone plays up communications. Dialogue. Rapport. But where does it get you?"

Many young people are able to shift responsibility to the circumstances surrounding a bad experience. "You want a bad trip?" says one boy. "You get this rotten stuff in some gin mill, which you can't leave because you're in someone else's car and a hundred miles from nowhere. So you get sick and puke all over your shirt and then have to stand the smell and clammy feeling for hours."

How does heavy drinking in the family affect young people?

Frequently, a discussion on booze will focus on other family members who drink too much and whose influence is felt strongly by the speaker. The following dialogue is from a teen rap session:

STEVE: Everybody seems to start getting drunk at sixteen. What's your attitude toward alcohol, Lill?

LILL: I try to stay away from it. I don't want to become a drunkard. My foster father was a drunkard and I didn't like him. I don't think people would like me if I was a drunk.

STEVE: What was it like living with someone in the family who was drinking all the time?

LILL: You never knew what would happen. He'd come home sometimes. He'd fall down sometimes. And he'd talk to the dog. The way he talked, the poor dog would get scared stiff.

SHAWN: That's nothing much to worry about. You should see what happens when someone gets the hates when he drinks.

TONY: You mean the "shakes"?

SHAWN: No, hates. H A T E S. My father is one of the good guys when he's sober. But he has a few boilermakers and he turns into a gorilla. He hates everyone. He's gotta fight, curse. He's a real Dr. Jekyll. Liquor can do mean things to a guy's system.

MIA: What happens in my family is that my mother doesn't drink because she gets ill. But my father does, and he's unpredictable. Sometimes he's smiling and happy—other times he picks a fight. When he's mean I leave the house. Sometimes my mother goes out with me. Most of the time she stays and doesn't listen to him. She may tell him the next day how he acted, but he won't believe it.

DUKE: My father used to drink, but not any more. He got so he wasn't getting to work on time. He'd always argue with us and sometimes make like he was going to sock me if I didn't agree. But he knew better because I was bigger and could clobber him. But now he's been on the wagon and sober a year. When I drink, I never do it at home, unless he's not there. It really isn't fair to drink in front of someone who's off the sauce—except alcoholics who've been in A.A. a long time and say they don't mind.

The question was asked at another rap session, "Would you like to be the same kind of drinker your father is? or your mother?"

DUKE: Count me out.

MIA: No way.

STELLA: My stepfather, I think he must be an alcoholic. I don't want to be like him. And my mother, she doesn't drink much during the week, a beer or so. On the weekends she gets plastered. I don't want to drink, to be like either one of them. I'd like to take a drink every once in a while, when there's an occasion.

MEG: My father drinks and my mother doesn't, and he follows her around and slaps her sometimes. My sister and I step in and slap him right back and he stops. He knows how we feel, but that doesn't seem to make him let up. I have a girl friend and we can go to her house and sleep over whenever we want. But sometimes my mother won't leave home. She's a bug for punishment and afraid the old man will injure himself or set fire to the house. He's very careless with the butts.

Do you set a good example in your own drinking behavior?

"Not infrequently," commented the director of one alcohol-education program in Ohio, "parents betray such questionable drinking habits themselves that they can hardly offer any advice about alcohol without evoking laughter or disbelief. Hence they find it preferable to stay in the shadows, maintain silence, and hope that their sons and daughters will come out better than they did."

Looking at it positively, and assuming that most parents who drink are moderate in their habits, reasonable guidelines can be followed in the home and community that will influence young people more by example than by regulation. The following suggestions have been mentioned frequently by educators and counselors in the field of alcoholism:

• Don't glamorize drinking by describing exotic drinks and potent cocktails that offer a 90-proof escape from reality.

• Be careful about expressing the need for a drink to neutralize fatigue, anxiety, or frustration.

• Avoid associating alcohol with rewards for hard work, success, or personal endurance in completing some arduous assignment.

• If it is natural to your life-style, feel free to associate wine and spirits with pleasant occasions, such as family dinners, engagements, or friendly get-togethers, but don't put more emphasis on drinking than on good fellowship.

• If you are a teetotaler, be tactful in trying to influence young people to practice abstinence. There are too many tragic cases in which young people have reacted so adversely to pressure and threats that they have gone in the opposite direction and become problem drinkers.

• Without forcing the issue, make it clear that drinking beer can have the same end result as consuming hard liquor, and that wine can sneak up on a person with sad results.

• Be wary of the trap many adults are getting into these days: encouraging drinking over smoking pot as the lesser of two evils.

• For cocktail parties and other occasions when you serve alcoholic beverages, make sure that there are plenty of non-alcoholic refreshments for those who do not want anything stronger.

• Never try to push a drink—even a beer—on a guest. Offer it, if you will, but only by letting the guest know what is available.

• If you prepare mixed drinks, measure the ingredients as carefully as you would for a favorite recipe. Have a bartender's guide handy if you are at all unsure of yourself.

• Keep liquor out of sight, not sitting on counter tops and open bars where it seems always to invite instant use.

• Don't make a habit of having the refrigerator always well stocked with beer and highball mixes.

• If you use alcohol, drink in the same manner you would hope to see your children adopt—because that is probably just what they will do as they unconsciously pick up your habits, good or bad.

What must parents know about alcohol?

Many adults tend to shy away from such knowledge, figuring that the less they know the less likely there is to be a problem. But look at the matter as realistically as you would any subject relating to health and well-being. Do most parents know anything about alcohol and health? alcohol and sex? the effects of different drinks on the body? What happens to the nervous system after the ingestion of six ounces of whiskey? What about the nature of alcoholism, the disease? Do they know that alcohol is a drug, and a depressant at that?

Probably not. With so much to learn about the glamorous and exciting side of alcohol, why bother with those dreary clinical facts?

One of the obvious problems is that only a handful of parents are personally endowed with the qualities they hope for in their children, and most parents are somewhat lacking in their own education concerning alcohol and drugs. Down through the decades and generations, we have grown up among as many myths concerning the subject as we have dandelions in the front yard.

Can you get high on aspirin and Coke? It was a popular belief back in the 1940s. Many adults will still swear that this is true.

How about bananas? If you lived in San Francisco in 1967, you probably heard the news that smoking banana peels, dried in the oven and then powdered, would produce vivid hallucinations. The only hallucination was "banana pot" itself, a real put-on.

Apple seeds. Green tea. Catnip. Celery leaves. Can these make you as high as a martini? Parents hear about them and are not sure.

Relax. They are just fads. But how is a parent to know? Sniffing glue was thought, for a brief period, to be a harmless pastime indulged in by small boys making model airplanes. Not so. It turned out to be highly toxic, the cause of hallucinations (real ones this time), slurred speech, depression, brain damage, and sometimes death.

What is your own attitude about drinking?

Traditionally, alcohol is consumed habitually, regularly, and in some quantity by the Italians, Spaniards, Greeks, Chinese, Lebanese, and Orthodox Jews with few problems and a low percentage of alcoholism. "It is important to note," says a report from the National Institute on Alcohol Abuse and Alcoholism, "that these major cultures, with long histories of relatively safe drinking, share certain common practices in their use of alcohol." The following are specially noteworthy for parents who drink and who have teenagers who are—or might be—into drinking:

- The parents themselves are consistently moderate drinkers.
- Beer and wine are the alcoholic beverages most commonly served in the home.
- Such drinks are usually taken with meals.
- Moral values are not associated with drinking; it is neither a sin nor a virtue.
- Those who wish to abstain on any occasion, or on all occasions, are never pressured to have a drink.
- Drinking is not viewed as any kind of proof of maturity or virility; in fact, children are exposed to it early in life.
- Neither drunken behavior nor excessive drinking is ever condoned, no matter what the occasion.
- The etiquette of drinking properly is taught early in life and observed by all ages.
- Drinks are sipped for enjoyment, not gulped for the effect.
- New types of drinks are seldom served; the participants invariably drink beverages with which they are familiar.

What is a reasonable guide to follow in teaching children about alcohol?

No matter how much information and counsel an adolescent may receive in an alcohol education program at school, through a youth group, or by some other organization outside the home, the basic responsibility almost always lies with the parents: how they act as well as what they say. "One cannot counsel a child with wisdom," advises the Utah Alcoholism Foundation, "until having examined one's own attitude toward alcohol with total honesty. This is the first step.

"The next step is to decide what attitude you want your boy or girl to take toward liquor.

"The third step is to help your child develop a good attitude toward alcohol and live by it."

A national youth organization that is deeply concerned with programs on alcohol abuse and prevention is Boys' Clubs of America, which has drawn on many sources to establish communications guidelines, based on advice from educators, psychologists, and specialists in the field of medicine and health.

Here are some tips for parents published in one BCA newsletter under the heading, "Straight Talk about Alcohol":

You drink? Talk freely and openly about what you drink and why you drink (even though it may seem obvious that they already know). If you or other adults in the family drink too much, be frank about that problem, too.

You don't drink? You are in a better position than parents who do drink to guide your children in the direction of abstinence. But do not use this abstinence on your part as a club to force your children to be teetotalers.

You have drinking habits? Think about them and determine what you are teaching by example. Do you urge drinks on guests? Do you look on mild drunkenness as humorous? Do you sometimes assert that you *need* a drink?

You abstain and have no drinking habits? But how about your nondrinking habits? Do you overplay the role of teetotaler? Do you rant about drinking as some form of evil? Or nondrinking as evidence that you are a "good" person? Think about your attitudes and actions from the viewpoint of young people.

You want to introduce your children to alcohol the right way? Do so first in the home, preferably at meals, so they view it as a normal part of life, not an end in itself. Distinguish between commonplace use, such as having wine with dinner, and special occasions, such as punch at Christmastime or sparkling wine on an anniversary.

You do not want to overreact? You read the horror headlines and are inclined to panic. Don't get trapped into thinking that dramatizing the dangers of alcohol will prevent young people from drinking. It failed to work with drugs.

You want to present the facts? Talk frankly about alcohol use and abuse in terms that relate to your community, your family, your children. Many adults fall prey to statistical thinking, and cite nationwide figures and surveys. In most cases these are meaningless to families and individuals.

You worry about teenage peer pressures? Think about your own peer pressures—friends, relatives, and neighbors who sometimes urge you to do (or not do) things. Teenagers are more susceptible to such pressures because they do not have the experience or convictions to resist comfortably. Arm your children with some logical reasons for not drinking—ones that are firm and reasonable, not just excuses. ("I'm not drinking today" or "I'm all set for now, with a Coke, thanks" are more effective than complicated stories.)

You feel uncomfortable talking about alcohol? You should not feel this way if you orient yourself with the basic facts about drinking and young people. There is no need to think about alcohol as something to be discussed in secret.

You dislike the aura of glamour around alcoholic beverages? You may feel that it is difficult to hold a heart-to-heart discussion with a young person and compete with the "in" look that beer, wine, and liquor have in magazine ads and TV commercials. Don't try to compete; *most* products are overglamorized in ads and commercials. Talk directly about what concerns you.

You want your adult viewpoint to be understood? If you expect your viewpoint to get a hearing, make sure you give the same kind of hearing to the viewpoint of a young person.

You want to get to the point and get the discussion over with? It is better to have no discussion at all than one in which you do rapid-fire talking and try to get instant agreements. Listening is vital; a good, leisurely rap session that reaches no startling conclusions may open up the way for future discussions and a better rapport and sense of understanding.

You have already drawn your conclusions? Scrap them, or at least hold them in abeyance and rethink the issues at hand. Your conclusions may be based on isolated statements, misinformation, or bias.

You're afraid you'll make mistakes? Everybody is going to make mistakes. Admit that you do not know all the answers and in some cases you know only part of the answer. Make it clear that a person is not "dumb" because of a lack of knowledge—only if he tries to pretend that he knows it all.

You get too emotional when you discuss sensitive and personal issues? So do most people. Treat that as a natural part of the dialogue and respect any emotional response on the part of your child. But never let the emotion itself become an issue.

You feel that the situation is beyond your control? If you have tried to establish a dialogue without success, or find that talking seems to be getting you nowhere, seek professional help. There is no need to look upon this alternative as a sign of weakness or failure, any more than if you called in a specialist to diagnose and treat a stubborn illness.

5 | Do adults practice what they preach?

Older people are often astonishingly insensitive to the reactions and impressions of young people when it comes to drinking. They seem to feel that there are two standards, one for adults, the other for youth.

The director of an alcohol education program for the sixth and seventh grades described a dinner that about a dozen of her pupils had been invited to attend. Several speakers were scheduled to discuss alcoholism before a group of doctors. Unfortunately, there had been a lengthy cocktail party beforehand and by the time the pupils arrived it was evident that several of the doctors and their guests had imbibed too freely. The wife of one physician decided to play the role of greeter, which she did gushingly and a bit sloppily, with many comments about how she had four lovely children of her own and they were not involved in anything as dreadful as alcohol. The fact that she was never seemed to enter her mind.

"The kids sized her up the minute she appeared on the scene," said the counselor later. "She made an ass of herself, as did one doctor who kept informing anyone who would listen that the idea that alcohol destroys the brain cells is sheer nonsense. He had been drinking for years and was still alert and brilliant."

As the meeting broke up, the young guests were treated to the spectacle of a gray-haired man arguing with his wife who was worried that he had polished off too many drinks to drive home safely. One of the pupils summed up the experience aptly when he reported later in a classroom session "I'm not sure that I understood the speakers too well because they used

35

a lot of medical terms. But I *am* sure that we all learned a lot about alcoholism."

This may seem to be an extreme case of how adolescents are turned off by adults—yet it is so only in the numbers of people and examples involved. Many a parent who drinks too much on occasion can recall instances in which he has exposed his children to garbled speech, or arguments over who should drive, or thick-tongued reassurances that he has not had too much to drink.

How do people learn to drink?

"Drinking is a learned behavior," says a report covering the first two years of the Cambridge and Somerville Program for Alcoholism Rehabilitation (CASPAR) in Massachusetts. "Drinking is learned by watching parents and other adults. Many young people have never been exposed to responsible drinking; or if they have been, have not identified it with drinking at all, which they regard from most of their observations as getting drunk—a view long recognized as a seedbed for alcoholism.

"In too many homes what kids are learning is irresponsible, or sometimes alcoholic, drinking. The two salient points are, *first,* that people learn about alcohol and drinking one way or another, whether the information is useful or dangerous, correct or incorrect; and *second,* that the lack of an aggressive attempt to foster positive learning leaves the field free to the many sources of negative learning."

For example, one teenager said, "I can't drink without getting freaked out. My mother, though, she sips *naranja* liquor she makes herself. It is a good thing for her. Also for my grandmother who lives at our house. With six small kids, you know she might go bananas if she doesn't have a little *naranja* now and then. Like a medicine."

Do parents sometimes demand too much?

Authoritarian parents can be described as those who demand certain types of performance and who give orders without explanation or provision for open dialogue. Often the children of such parents feel unrespected as individuals, or sense that they are not loved or understood. They may be subject to mistrust, shame, doubt, and guilt, and lacking in self-control, drive, and motivation.

"Defensiveness and a sense of insecurity on the part of parents and other significant adults in the family," explains counselor John Zachariah of Rochester, "do not foster proper communication and relationships." Uncomfortableness on the part of parents in dealing with a behavior they themselves have perpetrated, interferes greatly in establishing communication. "In some cases, alcohol use by children was interpreted as threatening the adult authority and defying their power."

There is also, Zachariah says, confusion about drinking—based on age (legal) and moral/ethical standards. Rebellious attitudes and unacceptable behavior often result when parents set high ethical standards for their children that do not jibe with adult drinking behavior. Because of the conflicting messages adolescents receive, some children conform to the adult drinking behavior out of a need to identify with the people who play significant roles in their lives. Unfortunately, he found this common among children of alcoholic parents.

In some cases, Zachariah reported that drinking was a form of self-destructive behavior which young people acquired as a direct means of getting attention and seeking help.

Many parents are not aware of the actual influence they have on young people. Professional counselors agree that teenagers are drinking in a way that could lead to alcoholism later and that the way they use alcohol is influenced by patterns established by adults. Parents must be firmer in laying down rules for the use of alcohol and in setting the right tone.

When young people attend a function where they are torn between the parental urge not to drink and the urge from peers to have a drink, there is no doubt that peer pressure can be a strong factor.

A young woman described the development of her drinking problem, which was stimulated by peer and family pressures, as well as her father's alcoholism.

BABS: Maybe I could have coped with Dad's drinking, thinking, you know, that my dad's head wasn't screwed on quite right and he didn't realize he was doing one thing and thinking another. My real problem was that our religion doesn't condone any kind of drinking, or smoking either. My mother told me it was a sin to drink. My boyfriend gave me a beer and I really liked it. But the smell was a giveaway and I used to suck mints and spray lotion to hide the smell before I went home. It made me more and more edgy and I finally *had* to have drinks at parties to enjoy them. Then I discovered that vodka didn't leave much odor and, well, you know . . .

LOU: Right. The guys I know who can't handle booze are mainly the ones whose old man is strict and says he'll restrict them or cut off their allowance if they ever drink.

How do parents foster irresponsible drinking behavior?

One teenager expressed the situation very well when he described it to some fellow students during a discussion on booze:

ARNIE: My father used to drink but he never acted drunk. Every night when he came home the first thing he'd do after he took his coat off was just go into the bar, take his Pinch out of the cabinet and pour it over ice, and sit down and have a drink and read the newspaper. My mother'd get the dinner while he sat there drinking. And you know, he could go to bed and the next day go to work and then come home and drink, same thing day in and day out. My sister claimed he was an alcoholic. There's a difference between being an alky and just a steady drinker. I think that the difference is if you're drinking day in, day out and you *must* have the drink or go bananas, then you're alcoholic. I never drank a lot myself, but once in a while I'd go overboard and get drunk. The first time I ever drank was at my uncle's house. He asked me if I wanted anything to drink and I said, "No, because I don't drink." Then my father pulled a switch with the glasses, so I ended up with his whiskey and he ended up with my gingerale. When I took a gulp I found out what happened. You know, it wasn't too bad. I did choke a bit that first time and after that I just drank a little bit now and then.

I won't drink whiskey anymore, and I don't drink beer. I drink vodka and that's it. My mother and father used to have a bottle of wine on the dinner table five nights out of seven. I could never pick up a taste for wine, not even champagne. Lot of times I won't drink. But sometimes you get pushed into it. Like this time in Maine. I was up there with a friend and his wife and they set me up with this chick who went along. And we drank a little bit. They told me that in Maine if you don't drink it's very, very unsociable. That's mostly what they do up there, everybody. They're real heavy guys, all seamen, with the idea "I'm gonna go out and get drunk!" We went to this night spot and everyone was drinking heavily. Even the band was getting into it. Every time my friends ordered, I ordered a round. Next day I woke up and I wasn't where I was supposed to be. I thought I was hanging from a tree, swinging. One thing had led to another and I don't remember . . .

Do parents practice a double standard?

"You can take the car when you have a date," says Roger M., a concerned parent who has been impressing on his eighteen-year-old son that in 50 percent of the auto accidents in which there are fatalities the driver has been drinking, "but do not ever drive it after you have consumed alcoholic beverages."

Roger M. and his wife always take the car when they go off to cocktail parties in the evening. The next morning the car can invariably be found in the driveway, even though Roger may stumble down to breakfast, grousing that he feels a bit hung over. Roger always drives the car home. And his son knows it. If he were questioned about it, the father might say, "I drove very slowly—we were only nine blocks away," or, "I had two cups of strong, black coffee before I left the party."

Do young people resent this bias?

Some comments were recorded at an alcohol workshop attended by high school students near St. Louis. All of the young participants had been having problems with booze. Two were recovering alcoholics. The group leader was a member of Alcoholics Anonymous in St. Louis.

CARL: I got some privileges taken away because I was out after one o'clock on a Saturday, maybe a half hour later than I said I'd be home. "It wasn't the hour," said my pop, "it was that you went to a beer blast at ten and here you were three hours later still into the suds." You know, he and Mom go to a cocktail party— drinking whiskey or gin, not just beer—and they think nothing if it lasts three hours.

BERNIE: My parents made a big thing over the "legal" angle,

that when I was drinking I was underage and breaking the law. But for a while we lived in a town that was "dry" and yet there were all kinds of ways people could get drinks—adults could, anytime they wanted. The law is one thing to adults and something else again to youths.

RHODA: One of my friends got high and was being a mimic and really funny. My mother got really annoyed and said I should go out with friends who were more mature. But just a couple of days later my mother was watching a TV show. It was a dumb show, in which a middle-aged lady was getting tipsy at a wedding and making an ass of herself and my mother thought it was hilarious. My friend had been much funnier. Why this kind of double image?

KAREN: My father comes home from work and pretty often says, "Boy, I really need a drink!" and he gets out a beer or mixes a cocktail. So he works hard and I'm sure he needs a little relaxation. But he heard me say that one time, after we had a tough exam period and it was all over but waiting for marks, and he chewed me out—as much as though I had said something insulting to my mother. But he keeps right on saying the same thing, "Boy, do I need a drink!"

ABE: I don't drink any more, but when I did, my father used to tell me all the time that I was drinking too much, or I'd had enough to drink. He was into the bottle a lot, too. But if I ever said he was loaded, he would've beat me up. He did, too, a couple of times.

TRISH: My mother puts marks on the liquor bottles so she can tell how much is used up. She admits she does it because my two brothers, nineteen and twenty, drink on weekends. I don't think that's a very mature way of doing it. Can't she trust us? It's almost like opening our mail.

BUZZIE: My mother and father are pretty fair about drinking, and I'd say realistic. But I don't like the way some of their friends act, who are in their forties or so. If we are at a family party, like around Christmastime, and have a drink in our hands, they feel they have to make some kind of remark, as though we couldn't drink very well socially.

MOOSE: How about adults who are always popping pills— tranquilizers, sleeping pills, or a shot of brandy to help them relax? These are the ones who then turn around and call a guy a dope addict because he has puffed a little grass. Who do they think they're kidding!

Kids who gripe about one set of standards for adults and

another for youth generally have a valid reason for feeling that way. "I think there is a definite double standard in drinking practices," says Eddie McNees, outreach coordinator for the Mid-Cumberland Council on Alcohol and Drugs in Nashville, Tennessee. "In the Bible Belt many fundamentalist churches preach that drinking alcohol in any form is a sin. Many times one parent will be teaching the children that drinking is sinful while the other parent is drinking excessively. This type of occurrence plays a definite part in the child's life."

As several other counselors have expressed it, young people react very negatively when parents or other adults try to inflict the double standard on them—"Don't do as I do, do as I say."

Teenagers and adults can develop more positive attitudes that will help both groups go through life handling beer, wine, and alcohol in a sensible, largely problem-free manner. Timmy, a member of "Choosers," a group of young people in Alcoholics Anonymous (A.A.) who are recovering alcoholics and who meet regularly twice a week, answered this question: "Booze has been such a bad scene in your life. How should drinking be handled by parents and children in order to avoid, or at least minimize, the problems that brought you into A.A.?"

TIMMY: Mainly I'd say that parents have to be careful not to set up a double standard. My old man is the first guy to head for the bar at a party, and the last one to leave it, but all I had to do was to look at a beer and he'd slap my ass.

What is the influence of the media?

Dr. John C. Heffelfinger, a specialist in the field of alcoholism, says of alcohol abuse among teenagers, "Our biggest problems are parents and television. We've become an alcoholic society, so alcohol is going to be used and abused because it's our standard way of living."

Gary Fair feels that "Hollywood and television have brainwashed us over the last twenty years to believe that we are not to have one unpleasant moment or endure a minute of pain. We are daily bombarded with the idea that drugs and alcohol will keep us well, make us beautiful . . . rich . . . and famous."

But is it all TV and Hollywood? Not necessarily. Fair cites an article in a professional journal that told about a group of psychologists who were asking drug companies to assist them in a project to find a sedative with no side effects. It was to be used to alleviate the trauma of children's first day in kindergarten!

Since there is immense confusion in the adult world about drinking and drugs, it takes little imagination to picture the conflict in the mind of the young person who is trying to understand the pros and cons, shape an attitude, and step forward in the right direction. Frequently, adults are unaware of the contradictions that children constantly see. Consider the irony of this everyday experience:

Although liquor commercials have been banned from TV, children observe an enormous consumption of alcohol when they watch the dramatic programs on the screen. A column entitled "The Booze Tube," by Nicholas Johnson, published in an alcohol foundation newsletter, described the situation this way:

The average American consumes 182 gallons of liquid a year: 56 gallons of water, 32 gallons of coffee, 24 gallons of milk, and—well down the list in eighth place after tea, fruit, and vegetable juice—perhaps one or two gallons of liquor.

Now ask yourself: When was the last time you saw somebody drink a glass of water on television? It doesn't happen often. No, TV drinkers are a long way from real life. The disproportion in their consumption of liquor over water, compared with the ratio in real life, is 264 to 1.

Unfortunately, many of the characters portrayed on television seem to need a drink to alleviate or escape from their problems, to tough it out when facing the odds, to "make it" with dates, or to set up a hilarious comedy routine. No one knows what pressure such programs and sequences may bring to bear on young people and their drinking habits. Even if we did have statistics on a regional or nationwide scale, the impact might be less than meaningful to you. It's what your own teenagers are exposed to, in the home or elsewhere, that counts—but only as one more factor to be considered in your overall appraisal of the situation and your decisions about the steps that should be taken.

Does advertising promote youthful drinking?

Despite the people who laugh at the overdramatized commercials or scorn the cute names being created for alcoholic concoctions, there is no doubt that advertising has some influence on the pattern of drinking among young people. One youth workshop expressed strong reactions to the subject when asked the question: "What effect do you think media have on drinking and alcoholism in young people—the newspapers, TV, radio?"

ALAN: The beer commercials have a corner on the market. Kids don't read the ads in magazines, or get hyped up by them. So beer is it. Suds. They can look pretty cool to kids. *In,* I mean.

COUNSELOR: How about the advertising of liquor distributors who are selling chocolate-flavored drinks that contain alcohol? or those sweet wines?

STEPH: Those jokers are knocking themselves out trying to peddle liquid candy. Who goes for it? Maybe some small kids.

COUNSELOR: Do you think that youngsters, say around fourteen or fifteen, are encouraged to drink by those beer commercials? Especially the ones that feature famous athletes or other familiar personalities?

MARIO: Beer commercials show people who are great, handsome, with a lot of "gusto." They make the beer look like some health tonic. The people who drink it are physically fit, having fun, doing things. Real machos. These are the guys and gals who have it all put together. To a little kid, this is a magic transformation. He can't wait to start drinking beer.

I used to think of gusto as something healthy, out-of-doors, enthusiasm. Now all I can think of is this magic facade you have when you drink beer. Look what you have in many commercials: the big athletes who are popping open the cans and drinking. A little kid who sits there like he's handcuffed to the screen, staring at these heroes, also sees a bunch of drinkers. And the kid who is older and near drinking age—that's what beer drinking has got to mean to him, one way of being a hero.

COUNSELOR: Is drinking considered a symbol of affluence and sophistication?

KIRK: Sure. You want a good thing going? You're in this great restaurant and you have a new girl and your old man likes her, too, so he's given you enough bread so you can buy a steak and offer her cocktails and wine as well.

LISA: Uh huh. Even if the girl doesn't drink, she likes the offer. And the guy can't get loaded because he doesn't have enough (money). You could say it adds something to going out—dining out —on a date to see a real bartender mixing up proper drinks. Not some creep ripping everybody off with slugs of booze he's pouring at someone else's party where he doesn't have to pay the tab.

6 | *How do drinks affect young people?*

Dr. Ross Fishman of the National Council on Alcoholism spends a considerable amount of his time on the educational scene, talking to students of all ages. A panel of young people appeared with him on a Channel 5 (New York City) "Midday" television program.

"I didn't know tequila was much stronger than beer," admitted one of the teenagers being interviewed. "I thought I'd have a good time, laugh a lot, and be cool, have fun. But then you have to pay for it."

Another participant told how she and her cousins were so ignorant of the alcoholic content of wine that they used to have contests to see who could race through a bottle the fastest. Then all of a sudden—bang!

"They're going to fry their brain cells!" is the way one participant on the panel described what would happen to his slightly younger peers if they did not learn at an early age that alcohol can be potent and dangerous to those who do not have the knowledge to respect it.

Some teenagers at an overnight conference tried to untangle the nature of alcohol and the consequences of using it unwisely.

"Quick, everybody," shouted the group leader, "as I point to each of you around the circle give me a comment—one brief but meaningful conclusion to the words, 'When I drink, I . . .'"

GAYLE: Feel sleepy.
GRIFF: Think slower. More slowly.
DUKE: Time doesn't matter.

45

MARY: I only drink wine or beer.
COLETTE: I drink very little.
TERRY: It makes me silly.

After some of the negative effects of drinking were aired, a participant asked the question, "But drinking *can* be fun, can't it?"

GROUP LEADER: For a healthy person, not uptight with problems, a highball or two, or cocktails, can be relaxing and in a sense "fun." But the hitch is the person has to know his limits. He can have whiskey or beer or wine and feel good. Then if he stops, the depressant effect that comes later is not severe enough to upset him, physically or mentally.

BETH: How do you know when you've had "enough"?

GROUP LEADER: You can recognize when you've had enough and are losing control. If you don't, relatives or friends will let you in on the secret, if you'll listen.

Now, if you don't learn the simple facts about what alcohol is and how different types of alcohol affect people, you're going to . . . well, what do *you* think will really happen?

TONI: You'll lose your health.

NORA: Look like a stupe.

ALDEN: Get busted by the cops.

GROUP LEADER: You're going to end up in trouble with the law, eventually. Did you ever hear of a "Green Lizard"? I hope not. It's made with hair tonic, to give you an idea of what some alcoholics will resort to. Someone said that alcoholic beverages make the drinker feel good. But why? Because they put the mind to sleep, shut out a lot of things, including certain miseries. Did you all know that alcohol was a drug?

YVONNE: It's a drug because it's an upper.

GROUP LEADER: No. You probably think of it as an upper rather than a downer because people get "high." Think a minute. When you start to drink, where do you feel it first? In what part of your body?

RAY: In your mouth, when you talk.

CHRIS: I get a kind of tightness across the back of my shoulders. Not a tightness as much as a tingle.

TERRY: In my head, like it's lifting up from my neck.

GAYLE: A pressed feeling all over my upper body.

ROSA: In my hands, down my fingers, especially the tips.

GROUP LEADER: How about experiences? Do you usually feel

good when you have a drink? Does that change to bad? Or mixed up?

RAY: Yeh, I always feel a good experience, even if I have too much and throw up. I always come out smiling.

DUKE: When I drink, I seem to do more. Maybe I don't really, but it sure seems that way. More activity, more talking, more experiences.

COLETTE: I can't drink wine. What does this mean? I drink wine and it makes me feel funny. It doesn't make me sick. My heart beats fast. I want to run.

GROUP LEADER: We have a lot of reactions here. Now what happens if you go to a party and drink until you're bombed?

RALPH: You pass out.

GROUP LEADER: Would you pass out if you weren't under the influence of a sedative drug? What happens the next day?

TED: You get a big headache.

DEAN: Hangover. All over, not just your swollen head. Your stomach, your guts. Sometimes you're dizzy and you can't stand up. But you can't lie down either because of that head.

NORA: One time when I drank too much I flipped out and was asleep for about twelve hours. But when I got up I was really faded. More tired than if I'd have stayed up all night dancing. Why?

RALPH: You use crazy energy. You keep going and going and going, but you really don't have as much in your battery as you would if you hadn't been drinking. Alcohol burns up your energy.

What is a hangover? One good answer is found in *Alcohol —Some Questions and Answers*, published by the Department of Health, Education and Welfare: *

A hangover is the body's reaction to excessive drinking. The associated miseries of nausea, gastritis, anxiety, and headache vary from case to case, but there is always extreme fatigue. No scientific evidence supports the curative claims for coffee, raw eggs, oysters, chili peppers, steak sauce, vitamins or other drugs, or the "hair of the dog." Doctors usually prescribe aspirin, rest, and solid food. If you choose to drink, the best way to avoid a hangover is to avoid drunkenness. Sip slowly, with food in the stomach, under relaxed circumstances, and pay attention to your responses to the alcohol so you don't drink too much.

---

* Available from the U.S. Government Printing Office. See Appendix: Pamphlets for how to order.

Where do marijuana and "getting high" fit into the picture?

At a rehabilitation center a number of young people were asked to discuss smoking pot, getting high on various drugs, and what the general teenage attitude is on these subjects. A counselor in his early thirties told the group that one of the big problems in the schools right now is the amount of alcohol being passed around. "We are more worried about alcohol than marijuana," he said. The teenagers had questions:

SCOTT: What if you had a son and he said to you, "I'd like to get high. Which way is better?" Would you let him get high?

GROUP LEADER: I'd say, "Get high *naturally*, without taking anything at all." By that, I mean I'd encourage him to enjoy normal feelings of joy and exuberance and uplift that young people can have when they are excited about something, or in love, or enthusiastic, or anticipating an event. You don't need a chemical—certainly not at your age—to be up in the clouds. But if I were to choose between pot and booze, I'd tell my son that alcohol is more dangerous. It has been proved to be extremely destructive to the human body.

DAVE: What's wrong with getting a buzz on from a few beers or a joint? I'm not saying to overdo it or get blasted, but just a nice glow?

GROUP LEADER: My attitude toward getting high has changed a great deal in the last few years. When I was in college everybody seemed to be getting high. I did, too. Then I decided that getting high with chemicals—pot, liquor, beer, whatever the chemicals were—was a waste of time. I was messing myself up and I don't like to be messed up.

ANDRE: How do you feel about it now, then?

GROUP LEADER: My advice to someone who's getting high a lot of the time is that he or she ought to determine *why* there is the need to get into this state. For instance, some kids may get drunk or spaced out because they cannot talk to either of their parents. Getting high is a cop-out, an escape.

WAYNE: I hear that all the time. Like "My old man won't listen to anything I say, so I might as well get loaded. What's the difference?"

GROUP LEADER: Kids get high because they cannot handle school. Or because there is continual fighting in the home. Let me ask you: What are other reasons for getting high?

SCOTT: A lot of guys smoke pot to show off.

WAYNE: They want to hang in with some cool kids, so they'll slug some booze or hit a weed.

SCOTT: Kids who are feeling down do it to get pepped up.

GROUP LEADER: All right, let's concentrate just on alcohol. Why do people your age drink? Fifteen- and sixteen-year-olds.

ROBERT: I'd say if someone our age is drinking, it's mainly to be cool, loose.

SCOTT: Kids go out with their gang, their buddies, to drink, mainly to hang in with the group.

JOHN: It's not because they like to drink. It's because they are having problems, with their families, or something else. That's what people drink about. It's the same with pot, but it's easier for people to go to a bar and get booze than to locate some pot.

WAYNE: You don't usually drink on your own, unless you're an alcoholic. You don't see many kids take a six-pack and beat it off somewhere and get loaded by themselves. But lots of kids take a joint and go off alone and get high.

SCOTT: You wouldn't be drinking in the morning before going to school. But I can see smoking pot.

GROUP LEADER: Let me ask the group a personal question. *Why* do you have to take alcohol or pot or other drugs to get high? Earlier I used the expression, a "natural high." It points to a lot of things that are fascinating out there in the nonalcoholic, the nondrug world. Why can't you get a natural high, being with people? Or doing things that are healthy and exciting?

MORT: You get high on drinks mostly because you tried it one time and it worked. You felt good. So you go right back to what made you feel that way. Myself, I can understand what you said about getting high on doing things. I like basketball, competition, sports, things like that. I can enjoy anything straight, you know. But it's what a guy knows that taking a drink or smoking pot—it's going to give you that reaction, that high. With sports, you don't always know what it will be like. How you going to make out? Maybe great. Maybe not so great.

ZACK: I like to play my guitar. I can do straight and enjoy it. But if I smoke a joint or have a drink *while* I'm doing it, that changes the experience. It may not be better, but it's *different*.

BARRY: It's not freaky. It's like you're out there in a boat sailing around and you sight some land and you want to go over and see what it is. You're curious. I mean, it isn't anything maybe any greater than other land, but it's new to you. It's different.

CRAIG: It's not different after a while. I quit drinking. I just quit, gave it up. I decided it wasn't doing anything for me. So I quit. I don't see much difference.

How do parents view alcohol versus pot?

The issue is not all that simple, explains counselor David J. Huberty. "Parents set one standard for themselves regarding the use of alcohol and a somewhat different one for their children. However, on another level, there is frequently far too much support for alcohol use by adolescents, with an unspoken reassurance to themselves that 'Thank God he is not on drugs!' "

"Alcohol use," says Huberty, who is coordinator of detoxification and halfway house services at the Central Minnesota Mental Health Center, "is largely accepted by parents in contrast to their fear and hysteria when some unfamiliar drug such as marijuana or pills is being abused. Parents *should* be hysterical when these unfamiliar drugs are being abused, but I also think they should be fairly hysterical when alcohol is being consumed by a thirteen-, fourteen-, fifteen-, or sixteen-year-old to the extent that it has become a noticeable problem."

It is not in the scope of this book to discuss at length the teenage use of pot. However, the subject has to be aired briefly since some parents consider alcohol less harmful than marijuana, even though it has been proven that alcohol can ruin the liver and have other serious consequences. Many parents have never tried pot; they fear that it might lead to other types of unacceptable behavior, and so they warn, "Don't experiment!" You see a lot of older people drinking and getting tanked and you know it is going to ruin them. Yet you don't see many people over thirty puffing on a joint.

A counselor in one session asked the question: "You feel that taking pot helps combat boredom. What if I were to ask which chemical your parents would rather have you use, pot or alcohol? Which would they prefer?

ROBERT: I'd say reefers. My mother knows what hurts you and she'd probably say pot before drink.

JOHN: Alcohol. My mother found out once that my sister smoked pot when she was little. If she knew there was any pot around the house now, she'd have a spazz attack. She threw my sister out of the house for it. But she lets me drink beer.

SCOTT: My parents would say, "If I find Scotty with either one I'll break his ass." But they'd probably prefer alcohol.

JEAN: Alcohol, because they're going to say, "Pot's going to mess you up. You're going to be on pot, then pills, taking hard stuff." It'll make you crazy—that's what they'd say.

WAYNE: Alcohol, because my mother thinks pot is a drug and you are going to get addicted to it.

JACKIE: If you asked my mother, she'd say "Neither." If you ask her about a reefer she'll start telling that you're gonna get addicted and you'll start taking dope and whatnot. She'll figure you'll go with the hard stuff.

Is it a choice of one poison or another?

These points are worth considering in any teenage conversation or rap session about alcohol versus pot. But keep the differences in mind. The legal aspects are decidedly different. In most states an older teenager can buy beer, wine, or hard liquor legally or can simply go to the refrigerator or liquor cabinet at home. But in buying other drugs, particularly hard drugs, a person of any age risks becoming involved with underground peddlers, the illicit "subculture," and runs the risk of incurring legal penalties, including going to jail.

When does social drinking get out of hand?

In a group discussion concerning the difference between social drinking and problem drinking, it was pointed out that there are certain trends that provide danger signals. For one thing, alcoholism seems to hit certain families harder than others. Studies have been made to determine whether alcoholism can, in fact, be an inherited disease. Young people are often confused about how to determine when a drinking situation is getting out of hand. The following comments indicate this kind of confusion and demonstrate that much more alcohol education is needed in our schools and communities.

OLGA: I don't understand about alcoholics. They can't drink without getting sloppy drunk. Then they give up drinking entirely. Are they still "alcoholics"?

CARLOTTA: They wouldn't get drunk if they were on the wagon, but they would still be alcoholics. It's still there—the alcoholism—because there's no way to treat it.

GERT: Can't alcoholics take a drug called Antabuse to combat drinking?

TONY: Yes, but it's not a cure. I tried some once. It just makes you puke and get real sick inside if you drink.

GERT: I passed out twice in my life and it was because I mixed drinks, and I don't ever want to have the curtain pulled down on me again. So I stick with beer or wine or soda. But my question is this: Is it a *blackout* when you pass out? What's a blackout?

BENNY: That's serious stuff. You're strictly into alcoholism—not just alcohol—when you have a blackout. You might pass out later, but a blackout is when you lose your memory. You may be walking around, laughing, telling some people to come on over to your house tomorrow for a party. And the next day you haven't the foggiest—you don't remember what was going on. So if a bunch of people show up and say, "Hey, Gert, here we are for the party you invited us to" and you draw a blank—sister, you've had a blackout.

GERT: How long does it take to get to that stage?

TONY: I knew this dude who never had a drink in his life. He came from some hick town out West where it was dry. No booze, not even beer. He got hooked on booze and in a year, maybe less, he was an alcoholic.

HELEN: I don't think it can work that fast. Not in a year, unless he had some kind of illness that maybe weakened his whole system. I've seen guys—kids and adults—go out on blasts practically every day and get smashed and keep it up for years before they are really alcoholics. The human system can take a lot of punishment before it caves in.

COUNSELOR: People's systems are different. Some do become alcoholics very quickly. I see this frequently in my own experience—kids who get to the problem stage real fast and others who drink a lot for a long time and never seem to change much.

SHAWN: The mother of a friend of mine is an alcoholic. Her husband travels a lot and she began to drink when he was away. No one seemed to know whether she drank because her husband was always away or whether he goes so much of the time because she drinks. This lady does have problems, though, and they could be the cause.

COUNSELOR: What do you think about a statement describing a woman—that she "drinks like a man"?

JOYCE: Women are becoming more like men in their drinking habits. Not our age so much as ones who are in their twenties or older. Women are going out and working like men. And they're drinking more like men.

STEPH: At home, though, women still have to take care of the kids and they don't always like the job and they start drinking to make life easier, or less boring. Or they have problems with the kids.

COUNSELOR: Are you saying that as alcohol becomes more socially acceptable to a group, then that group is drinking more? How does this relate to young people?

TONI: There is more drinking in high school, in all kinds of teenage groups, I think.

7 | How serious is the drinking problem?

"We are justifiably concerned about the effects of mind-altering drugs upon ourselves, our families, and our community," says New York counselor Dick McLaughlin. "We wonder when some drug will come along—let's call it Drug X—strong enough to destroy the fabric of our social, economic, and political structure through its widespread and devastating effects on individuals and communities. What would happen?

"Drug X is already here! What are some of its noxious effects, documented evidence of the Drug X pandemic in this country? Here are a few of the disintegrating effects it has already had on society:

"Ten million people, including increasing numbers of teenagers, have a dependence upon it that is out of control. Another 30 million are directly affected as close relatives of those afflicted.

"Users of Drug X are risking entry into a state of coma, but before that occurs they suffer impaired judgment, diminishing control over their behavior, severe reduction in physical control, and unusual proneness to accidents.

"Extreme aggressiveness as a result of impaired control has made X the most violence-producing of all drugs, accounting for some 90 percent of all assaults and more than 50 percent of all homicides.

"The suicide rate among those addicted to Drug X is six to twenty times higher than the rate in the general population.

"Drug X is directly responsible for hundreds of thousands of divorces, desertions, and separations, and it plays a key role in subjecting young children to neglect, persecution, violent beatings, and incest."

McLaughlin is not an alarmist. He is simply citing—as he often does—comments made in an alcoholism and drug newsletter that he distributes to students, teachers, parents, counselors, and others concerned.

Drug X, if you have not already guessed it, is *alcohol.*

Are many of our beliefs about alcohol really myths?

One of the myths most prevalent in the minds of young people is that alcohol is an aid to sexual prowess. Word quickly spreads around the school grounds when teenagers have achieved sexual conquests by plying their dates with drinks. Or when coeds have become pregnant because they had too much booze and went too far. Or when a boy who was usually shy and reserved finally managed to "make out" with his girl friend because a few beers loosened his inhibitions.

Sometimes parents are unwitting accessories to such seductions by setting their daughters up for the unwanted sequence of events. "Many parents are unduly anxious to see their children grow up," says Marvin Block of the American Medical Association's Committee on Alcoholism and Drug Dependence, "often to the point of pushing them into patterns of adult behavior before they are prepared for adulthood. . . . Drinking parties for high school students are anything but rare and too often are condoned by parents. Mothers who fear that their daughters will lack popularity and thus risk failure to make 'a good match' may rush them into adulthood long before they are prepared psychologically for such a role. Too often . . . the ambitions of the parents will lead them to approve drinking, if only as an attempt to enhance their children's opportunities, particularly if the children insist."

If a young girl is already beyond her depth because of this kind of pressure, or if she is subjected to an equally strong peer pressure to be "popular," she is not likely to have much judgment about drinking and how far she has to go to maintain her popularity. Thus, the stage is set well in advance, but the boys whose sexual advances are not rebuffed are likely to attribute the outcome to the magic stimulation of beer, wine, or liquor.

Under these circumstances, parents face a difficult, if not

impossible, challenge trying to convince teenagers—theirs or anyone else's—that Shakespeare was right when he wrote that drink "provokes the desire, but it takes away the performance."

In point of fact, drinking has a negative effect on sexual performance and, if carried to excess, can ultimately result in dysfunction and degeneration of the sex glands. Alcoholics often suffer sex problems, physiological as well as psychological. But this is not confined to chronic drinkers. A pathologist at Mt. Sinai School of Medicine in New York City, after studying the effects of alcohol on males, reported: "Anybody who drinks continuously can get the effect. This is a pure effect of alcohol in any form you take it—whiskey, wine, or beer. The total amount of alcohol is the only thing that counts."

Is a cold shower better than black coffee to put a drinker in shape for the drive home?

Mike Phillips is a driver education instructor at Central Catholic High School in Pittsburgh and an advisor for the Youth Traffic Safety Council of Allegheny County, Pennsylvania. He and his associates have promoted a public information and awareness campaign called SOBER (Slow on the Bottle, Enjoy the Road), to make young people aware of the dangers of drinking and driving. The school has also prepared a special "Driving While Intoxicated" course coordinated by teachers, the police, alcohol specialists, and probation officers.

Brother Mike gets through to his young students that neither showers nor coffee will do the job—only *time* can put a drinker back in shape.

Is it safe for you to drive a car if the alcohol content of your blood is less than the legal limit for arrest?

Just one drink will interfere with your reactions. And though your blood content may stay within legal limits, your chance of having an accident if you drive goes up in direct proportion to the percentage of alcohol in your blood.

Can counselors really explain what addiction is?

In this matter of kids and booze, there are more questions than there are answers. If you ever find yourself in the hands of a counselor or other professional who assures you that he knows most of the answers or has developed some kind of pet formula or theory that will put Humpty-Dumpty all back together again, beware! Gary Fair told me that one of the biggest problems in getting parents to understand alcohol is that they tend to over-simplify the issues. They want to set up some rules and guide-lines and have young people follow them. In trying to do so, they overlook dozens of factors that make it almost impossible to set up clear distinctions.

Having worked with persons suffering from alcoholism since 1963, Fair began writing an article on "The Addiction Dilemma" for a newspaper. Because of the complexities of the subject, it ended up as a series of almost a dozen pieces. As he points out, adults focus on the behavior problems that result from drinking, but are not at all clear about what excessive drinking can do to the health. "Increased drinking among teen-agers is becoming a major cause of malnutrition," he says, "even among youth with adequate food supplies. They face the same problems as an adult but, because of their inexperience and underdeveloped bodies, the destruction may be greater."

What are some of the effects of alcohol?

The adult who has been drinking to one degree or another over a period of years may think he knows the effects, based on his own experience. But so many factors enter into the situation that even the experts can never be completely sure what alcohol will do. Heavy drinking has as many "bad scenes" and "trips" as overdosing other kinds of drugs.

Just what is alcohol?

Dr. Ross Fishman of the National Council on Alcoholism pulls no punches. Alcohol, he says, is more dangerous than heroin. "When examining alcohol as a drug, it is important to see it within the larger context of drugs, as a sedative, hypnotic, or depressant." It is not digested like other substances. Instead of being broken down like other kinds of foods, it is absorbed right through the stomach wall into the bloodstream, whence it is distributed evenly throughout all the cells in the body.

"Alcohol has very small molecules, so it gets everywhere. The same amount of alcohol in people of different body weights is obviously going to have a different effect. . . . Therefore, one important factor is going to be the blood alcohol level and what that does to a particular individual."

Why does heavy drinking affect coordination?

Going through the bloodstream on the way to the brain, alcohol passes through the liver, which acts as a filter. If you drink only three quarters of an ounce of alcohol per hour, the liver can handle the load, changing it into water, carbon dioxide, and energy. Any amount more than that keeps passing through the brain, even after you stop drinking, until the liver has had a chance to carry out its function. The first area of the brain to be affected is the cortex, which coordinates body functions and involves motor coordination, thinking, and judgment. So when the cortex is depressed by alcohol, it loses its ability to control lower centers of the body.

You may get a tingling sensation in your fingers and toes. For some reason, booze tingles your extremities first, before it starts affecting other parts of the body. That is why people spill their drinks and slur their speech (the tongue is also an extremity).

Alcohol is potent, but is it lethal?

The Friday night "tapping" party at an upstate New York college was a common event, welcoming new pledges to an undergraduate fraternity. During the course of the heavy drinking that ensued, three of the pledges, in their late teens, became violently ill. Two were hospitalized in serious condition. The third died from a condition known medically as "diffuse pulmonary edema." In layman's terms, the young man had consumed so much alcohol that his system was not able to function effectively; he literally choked to death on his own vomit.

Alcohol can kill in many ways. It can be toxic. And between extremes, from a mild high to a DOA ("Dead on Arrival"), there are numerous variations on clinical conditions. Alcohol is *the* most abused drug. It can make you high, but it can also make you permanently goofy. It can eat away your stomach. A person with an ulcer should never drink because alcohol will make the tissues bleed. It can make your pancreas bleed as well. You may get sharp pains in the abdomen, vomit, and feel "seasick" all over.

How can alcohol make a person fat or bloated?

Alcohol is lacking in nutrients. It contains no vitamins, no proteins—just calories, which can help you on your way to a paunch, the common "beer belly." Many alcoholics suffer from malnutrition because they eat little or at best are on poorly balanced diets. In fact, if a person really drinks a great deal he can die from malnutrition—the combination of not eating much and eating improperly. Some alcoholics actually forget that they have not eaten, become extremely debilitated, and are susceptible to all kinds of illnesses.

Why does alcohol hit some people quicker and harder than others?

"I only had a couple of beers," says a teenager defensively when someone gets on his back for having made a fool of himself. Yet another youth may have consumed an entire six-pack by himself without giving evidence of being smashed. The difference may lie in the fact that the first youth chug-a-lugged his beers quickly while the second sipped his brew over a much longer period of time.

It is also commonplace for two people who consume the same amount of alcohol at the same speed to react in different ways—one seeming quite sober, the other a bit tipsy. Here are some of the factors that influence the effect of alcohol:

Weight. A person weighing 175 pounds has more blood and water in the body than the person at 110 pounds. The alcohol is more diluted in the heavier person and hence does not have as pronounced an effect.

Food. Alcohol makes its way into the bloodstream by passing through the walls of the stomach and intestines. Food in the stomach tends to retard the passage and lessen the consequences (up to a point).

Attitude. How a person thinks and feels can make a marked difference. If you drink purposely to get high, you are more likely to do just that. If you drink when you are sad or depressed or upset, you are likely to accentuate those feelings instead.

Location. Drinking with a convivial group increases your chances of feeling happy and "with it." Drinking alone sets you up for a mood of feeling sorry for yourself.

Experience. A young person unaccustomed to alcoholic beverages tends to show the effects of drinks more than a mature person who has been drinking for many years (in a nonalcoholic manner). The latter has become conditioned, perhaps subconsciously, to adjusting for the milder effects of booze in much the way a skier adjusts to higher altitudes or steep slopes, or a swimmer learns to breathe differently while in the water than on land.

Type of drink. The alcohol in beer and wine is more diluted than in hard liquor and is therefore absorbed more slowly into the bloodstream. Diluting liquor with water, fruit juice, or other noncarbonated mixers helps to slow the absorption rate. But mixing it with carbonated beverages can increase the rate, even though the same amount of alcohol is involved.

How much alcohol is there in a can of beer?

A can of beer containing twelve ounces of liquid has about one ounce of pure alcohol. That is the equivalent of the alcohol in a mild highball. A six-pack of beer is comparable in alcoholic content to three really stiff drinks of hard liquor.

Most kids, and many parents, either are not aware of the fact that beer has a substantial alcohol content or else they ignore it.

Do young people want advice from adults about drinking?

There is no ideal alcohol education program that will supplant parental influence or relieve parents of their responsibilities in dealing with sons and daughters who may have problems with alcohol or tendencies in that direction. Professional counselors and educators sometimes have communication difficulties, just like the rest of us. They encounter hard-core resistors who refuse to cooperate and skeptics who are constantly spreading doubt among other students. They often have inadequate facilities and limited hours for scheduling programs.

If you can sit in on an ongoing alcohol education program, you might learn a considerable amount about ways of communicating and getting through to young people in critical or highly sensitive situations. Leaping into the fray, prodded by the ultimatum "I've got to do *something!*" is seldom helpful. It might be of value instead to have an overview of the problems and alternatives facing professional counselors when they try to establish a meaningful rapport with young people, for both educational and therapeutic purposes.

How does a "dialogue" take place?

At a moderate-sized school in central Tennessee, where the community had been experiencing disruptions caused by undesirable, alcohol-related behavior, two professional counselors were assigned to see what they could do about such problems as destruction, noisy brawls, and beer drinking by young children. Eddie McNees, outreach coordinator, and Kathlyn Hatcher, training coordinator of the Mid-Cumberland Council on Alcohol and Drugs, worked with a group of twenty students, all volunteers.

The students were told that they could say *anything* they wished about alcohol and drugs and the two counselors would discuss it.

(This is a basic understanding that an adult should have with a youth, to make it possible to bring into the open those situations and problems that may have lain hidden because of an impression that they were too personal or too off-limits for discussion.)

Upon being told that there were no restrictions, no subject areas that were considered too sensitive for opening up, the students thought there must be some kind of a catch to the approach, something they should be wary of.

(A parent who has had very little, or very poor, dialogue with a son or daughter can logically expect to be eyed with suspicion if he unexpectedly announces that he wants to rap wide open on booze and related matters. It would be better to schedule some trial runs first, covering more restricted areas, before embarking on totally unknown seas.)

"I assured the students that everything mentioned in the session would be strictly confidential," says McNees, "and that they would be allowed to say whatever they wanted without fear of reprisal. There were to be no teachers in the group and I was not to discuss with any school official the dialogue of the sessions."

(Confidentiality and a promise of no disciplinary action are vital ingredients in any parent/child dialogue on drinking. Any adult who promises not to use what is learned in a session as a means of reprimand, and later violates that promise, will find the communication routes permanently blocked.)

Almost immediately, the students began quizzing McNees and Hatcher about their own experience with alcohol, marijuana, and other drugs. McNees countered by asking whether it was really important that the students know this and whether it was going to make any difference in the effectiveness of the sessions.

"If you don't drink alcohol or smoke pot, how are you going to be able to help young people who have problems with drinking or drugs?"

"Does a doctor have to have cancer in order to treat it?"

asked McNees. "Does a person have to have a broken arm to realize that it hurts?" The point was clear and the students gained confidence in their counselors.

(Young people, even in their late teens and early twenties, want to discuss problems with a person who has the necessary expertise and understanding. Too many adults have the mistaken impression that being a "parent" is enough of a credential to convince a young person that you have enough know-how to call the signals. Parents must be open and honest about what they know and don't know. Does this mean that a father who has never touched a drop in his life is totally unequipped to discuss problems with a teenager who has been high on alcohol on any number of occasions? Not necessarily. A *caring* parent can establish considerable rapport on a "Let's-explore-this-problem-together" basis, asking the child to think through the implications of his attitude and behavior. It is helpful, however, for the parent to have done some extensive homework on the subject of alcohol before committing himself to a one-on-one discussion.)

Early in the discussion, the students expressed resentment over the double standard practiced by many adults, that is, when they establish a different set of rules for themselves than they do for their children—not only when it comes to drinking but with regard to general life-style. A seventeen-year-old girl in the group described an occasion when her mother was waiting for her to return from a date. The mother immediately sensed that the daughter had been drinking, screamed at her, went into a panic, and then popped down two Valium pills to calm her nerves. The girl protested that taking the pills was just as harmful as her drinking three beers. But the mother's response was, "Go to bed. I don't want to talk about it!"

(This is a perfect example of the attitude that weakens the credibility of the adult, and makes it impossible to carry on a one-on-one discussion about drinking. While it is true that teenagers react differently than adults to alcohol for a number of reasons, this should not be stressed as a basis for setting up two different standards. The mother who drinks must accept the fact that her own recognition of alcohol as a beverage *implies* that it is part of an overall life-style in which her children also play a part. Age, legality, and inexperience are factors that naturally have to be considered, but the viewpoint should never be taken that it is totally right for an adult to drink and totally wrong for a teenager.)

One eighteen-year-old boy in the group admitted that the only thing he knew about alcohol was what he had learned from his peers and from experimenting for himself. Why had he not acquired any information from his parents? Because they insisted that "drinking is *wrong*," and that he must not drink.

"One of the problems we have faced in the past in dealing with alcohol and kids," says McNees, "has been the older generation telling the young people what they *thought* they should be told rather than listening and discovering what the young wanted to know themselves. Without exception, our students wished that their parents were more open about discussing alcohol. The group consensus was that parents tell teenagers not to drink, yet the only reason given is that 'It is wrong to drink.' This dictum is not acceptable to young people. Certainly it has not prevented them from drinking."

(Again and again, counselors have emphasized that adults are way off track when they play "right" against "wrong." Whether you drink a lot or a little, are a teetotaler, or have problems holding your liquor, drinking is an integral part of the overall American life-style, and of many other national life-styles. The ethnic groups, communities, families, and individuals who drink alcoholic beverages properly and without problems are the ones who accept beer, wine, or liquor as intrinsically neither "good" nor "bad," beneficial or harmful. In any objective discussion, behavior and attitudes are far more relevant subjects than the evils of alcoholic beverages.)

None of the students in the Tennessee volunteer group believed that they themselves had drinking problems, although every one of them admitted to having relatives or close friends who abused alcohol or were outright alcoholics. Most had been strongly affected by these relationships, as in the case of a sixteen-year-old girl who told the group that she did not drink at all because alcohol had ruined her father's life. "The hurt in her eyes was obvious as she talked about the relationship she now has with her father."

McNees strongly feels that one of the major problems of communication that must be overcome is the lack of trust in adults that is evidenced by many young people. "I do not know what causes this lack of trust," he admits, "yet I know that it is there. I see it in the way young people will deliberately test their parents, teachers, preachers, or any other adults to see if they are being honest with them.

"Sometimes kids ask adults questions for which they already know the right answers. If the adults who are victims of this kind of put-on are not honest, then they lose a trust that may take a long time—if ever—to regain. In working with teenagers, I have found that the one thing they demand from their families and friends is *honesty*. If that honesty is betrayed, kids will close the door between themselves and you—no matter who you are or how important you may be to them."

(Honesty includes the willingness of the adult to say "*I don't know*" when a question is beyond the reach of his/her knowledge or experience. The subject can be kept alive with the remark, "I really don't know. I wish that I did. But let's explore it together and see what we can find out.")

One of the significant findings of the rap sessions was documentation of the widespread viewpoint that alcoholism has been branded with an almost ineradicable stigma. Young people sense this strongly, though often because of parental attitudes. Members of the group readily admitted to knowing several "friends" who suffered serious drinking problems and whom they would like to help. Yet they always backed off and were unwilling to help the person find treatment because of a fear that the friend's parents would find out. "Although attitudes toward drinking are changing," says McNees, "we still have a long way to go. There are still many people who equate alcoholism with *a lack of will power*. Until teenagers feel comfortable with adults in dealing with friends or relatives who have drinking problems, they will continue to hide—or try to hide— the problems."

(Again and again counselors, doctors, educators, and other professionals have been emphasizing that alcoholism is a *disease*. You must accept this diagnosis if you are dealing with a young relative or friend whose drinking has gone beyond the stages of youthful experimentation or rebellion. If you cannot accept this interpretation, for whatever reason, you should seek the counsel of a professional in the field of alcoholism. You are going to need such help for the alcoholic in any case, so the sooner you seek it out, the better.)

One further problem area brought to the surface in the Mid-Cumberland project was what McNees and Hatcher pinpointed as a rebellious attitude on the part of some young people. They realize and readily agree that there are about 10 million alcoholics in the United States, that excessive drinking can increase the chances of heart disease, and that heavy drinking causes cirrhosis of the liver and other deadly diseases. Yet parents—also aware of these facts—continue to drink. At the same time, they become almost hysterical if they learn that a child of theirs has been puffing pot. The teenagers contend that there is no real medical proof that should influence them to stop smoking grass.

This is where the rebellion takes hold. Young people defy their parents on the grounds that adults *know* for a fact what the excessive use of alcohol can do, yet they continue to drink. They argue that if parents want to force their children to quit smoking grass because it *might* be harmful, they most certainly will have to quit drinking alcoholic beverages, which they *know* can be harmful. Part of the hysteria, of course, originates with the legal aspects of the matter, the knowledge that possession of marijuana can result in arrest.

"Whether it is a valid argument or not," says McNees, "that is the way many teenagers feel about the stand-off. The problem is that the door of communication is slammed shut and it may be difficult to pry open."

(Adults who have a problem talking with young people should try to avoid the booze-versus-pot controversy since it diverts the discussion from the basic problems. If it does come up, play it straight and admit that there are vital gaps in our knowledge, but try to steer the discussion back to the basics.)

Are attitudes as important as drinking habits?

This question was brought into focus when young people were asked how parents could best teach their children about alcohol.

CATHY: You have to influence them. A parent needs control. But you can't expect your kids to believe everything you say. You have to show them. One thing you shouldn't do is use any violence. It doesn't do much good to say, the way my father did, "Don't drink!" and "Drinking's bad for you!" and then let you see that he consumes plenty of drinks and doesn't follow the advice he tosses at you. My parents were rough, tried to force ideas down my throat to get me to conform, or not to do something, and it didn't work. I revolt whenever someone gets pushy. And it's downright silly for an adult to sit there drinking a cocktail and tell you not to drink because it's bad for you, even if you are too young.

BRUCE: Parents should never say to kids that they cannot go to a party simply because the parents are convinced some kids are going to get drunk. It doesn't help a kid any to be told he cannot go. If I gave my kid the car to go to a party and he got bombed and walked home, I'd tell him I was proud of him for making the decision not to drive. I wouldn't bug him for having gotten smashed. I might even say that *I'd* go back and pick up the car.

CATHY: He shouldn't be given all that much praise, since after all he did get bombed. I wouldn't knock him around, but I wouldn't praise him either. And I'd make *him* go back the next morning and pick up the car. Later, I'd talk to him and try to find out what happened. Not a confrontation. Just talking it through and keeping your cool.

COUNSELOR: What do you think goes on in the mind of a parent when a bad scene like this occurs for the first time?

TONI: "I'm a bad parent." That's what some will think. "I didn't handle this right or the kid wouldn't have gotten zapped." "Some of the other parents are going to find out what happened and then I'll be labeled Mr. Bad Parent."

MARIO: First of all, I'd want to know who the kid was out with. I'd ask what went on and I'd tell it like it was when I was that age, so we'd have a pipeline. Kids should be able first to see *concern* on the faces of parents. Mostly, they see the anger. And they shouldn't see that. Okay, so the parents are angry, but the caring is what's more important.

BRUCE: It's not all so much what the parent says as how he says it. He can say, "Now look, I'm worried about this because I *love* you . . ." And the very way he says it spouts anger—despite the words and the emphasis on love. That's not the right way. A father has to level with you that, look, I'm with you and I want you to be happy, and OK, but I'm worried about this kind of nonsense and what happened, and why, and whether we have a repeat performance.

STEPH: Let's say it's a young girl and probably the mother is the first to learn that her daughter has come home smashed and so she tells the father he's got to take a stand. It's *his* little girl. He's going to be under pressure from his wife to do something positive and preventive, as well as hassling over it himself and trying to figure what approach to take. The chances are he doesn't have the foggiest. If it's a boy, the whole scene is different. He's a guy and he can take care of himself, following a couple of strong remarks from the old man. And he can't get pregnant either. And so the crunch isn't as bad as with a girl.

EMMETT: I don't think you should treat them any different, whether it's a boy or a girl who's come home smashed.

CATHY: Let the poor kid know first that he or she is a good person basically, and that you—the parents—respect him. And if he's done this thing that's wrong, then talk it out. Don't start off with the idea that the kid is all wrong, a mess, and has to come up with excuses.

PAULA: I think parents should take a reasonable attitude and bring up children so they know what drinks are and how to handle them. Most kids, for instance, think it's OK to drink a beer. And another. And another. It's only four or five percent alcohol, or whatever. Same with wine—it's nothing compared with gin or rum or rye. That's what I thought and it's why I'm here. I guess my parents are kind of dumb. I don't blame them because *their* parents didn't provide much guidance. My mother would get worried about teenagers drinking at parties, but didn't know what to say in the way of advice. And Dad, he took the attitude that "Don't worry. It's only a phase. Let the kids figure it all out for themselves."

Are the problems of children all that important?

Eddie McNees says, "One of the major blocks is the fact that some parents don't allow children to make little decisions, and when the child is confronted with making a major decision, he does not know how. According to youths I have talked with, the problems and pressures each of them encounters are taken lightly by their parents, who seem to forget that young people growing up have experiences that are traumatic to them although the same experiences might seem petty to the parent."

McNees says that several young people told him that when they confided in their parents about something troubling them, they received this kind of answer: "Son, if that is the biggest problem you have, you are in good shape. Now, go on and don't worry about it. I'll take care of it." Consequently, when the day comes that the parents no longer handle such problems, the youth does not know what to do or whom to turn to. So sometimes he turns to alcohol, and when he relies on that to solve his problems they only become magnified. "If a teenager then develops a drinking problem," says McNees, "the parents, sadly, are the last persons to realize the truth."

How can you discuss drinking with a teenager?

In October 1977 the ABC television network broadcast a program called "Teenage Turn-On," which included several taped sessions of boys and girls openly discussing the problems they had encountered through the use of liquor and other drugs.

"Kids aren't just using one drug at a time any more," reported ABC. "Now it's deadly combinations of beer, pot, liquor, cocaine, and pills. And your children may be part of this enormous national problem without your even knowing about it. . . . Many parents are afraid to face the problem. But finding out in time can save you and your children a world of pain and heartbreak."

Elva Herzog, juvenile section psychologist with the Department of Police in Piscataway, New Jersey, feels that the biggest problem facing parents is that "they do not realize how to establish communications. They try to get children to stop drinking and end up in failure. What they need to know is that they would accomplish more if they would teach children *how to drink and when to drink*, rather than try to force them to abstain. They break the line of communication right away."

Gary Fair feels that "discussions at home between parents and young people would be more productive if the parents would only have the patience to listen to kids and not constantly accuse them of avoiding the subject." As he sees it, parents want to get right down to the subject (that is, if they have reached this stage of facing it at all) and talk in terms of specific actions. When did you drink? How much? How often have you gotten drunk? Do you intend to stop this behavior? And so on.

What they should realize is that an effective, meaningful dialogue can be a long and continuing process of talking and *listening*, not setting up or coming to agreement on rules and regulations.

"I never talk in terms of drinking and not drinking when I'm having a discussion with young people," says Fair, "but rather of the effects of alcohol, what it is and what it does. I'm interested in the comments of the kids about what it does to them, or what they think it does to others. This approach leaves it up to the listeners or participants to make up their own minds and puts no pressure on them to take my advice."

Is it important to be yourself?

If you are a parent or other adult trying to steel yourself for the ordeal of facing your teenager on "drinking," the best thing you can do is *relax* (but not with a drink!). "Don't feel that to reach young people you have to look like them, with a beard or jeans or rumpled hair," Fair advises. "Just look like yourself, wearing whatever is normally appropriate for you at that time of day and in that place."

This is not just talk. Gary Fair looks like what most kids would refer to as a "square." He generally wears a business suit, shirt, and tie when he meets with young people for discussions on alcohol, and young people seem to respect him for being himself. One recent session was with an all-black class, teenagers who had been described as "hard-core" because they were involved in so many drugs and booze. Fair appeared in his usual business suit and had a very satisfying encounter. Later the participants voted him the best, most interesting speaker they had listened to all year, and the one they could best identify with.

How should a parent go about beginning a dialogue at home?

Counselors and teachers suggest the following procedures and outlooks for parents contemplating confrontations with sons or daughters on practically any subject, but especially on alcohol:

- Be yourself and do not attempt to play some other role.
- Have plenty of patience and let discussions cover as much territory as seems necessary—short of changing to a completely unrelated topic.
- Don't let yourself be intimidated. If attempts are made, simply roll with the punches and continue the discussion.
- Never talk down to a young person.
- Don't try to speak in teenage jargon, except for words and phrases you normally use in conversations.
- Be honest, even blunt, in what you express. You rapidly lose credibility once you make statements or express opinions that seem forced or fabricated.
- Throw in enough pertinent facts to keep your credibility alive, but not so many as to confuse the listener.
- Do not take a righteous, I'm-older-and-I-know-better stance.
- Try to avoid being a bore.

A more concise set of guidelines was developed by the Cambridge and Somerville Program for Alcoholism Rehabilitation as four keys to effective teaching:

First, you must be clear about your own attitudes and feelings about alcohol in order to talk about it objectively, as a "neutral substance"—that is, one that is not in itself either "good" or "bad."

Second, you must set aside the time and have the patience to evaluate your own ideas about the way young people drink and think about drinking. Perhaps, like many adults, you do not give young people enough credit for being able to behave responsibly, with or without alcohol present.

Third, taking the realistic attitude that young people are capable of arriving at responsible decisions, you should be able to reach this responsible decision of your own: to avoid lecturing, preaching, occupying center stage, and otherwise inhibiting positive responses and discussions from teenagers.

Fourth, be careful how and where you place the emphasis in discussing alcohol and alcoholism. You do not need to stress the disease if you are simply trying to talk about alcoholic beverages and drinking patterns in the home and community.

How can parents initiate a rap session?

Perhaps it would be better to stay out of the picture, leave the responsibility to someone more knowledgable. After all, you probably don't try to teach science or a language to your children. So why a tough subject like alcohol and alcoholism?

Would you rather have your children attending a course that is inadequate? Maybe you should skip the whole thing.

These are some of the unsettling questions you may need to answer. For example, on investigation, you may find there is no adequate alcohol education program available in your community. You can start a campaign to develop a proper course of instruction from scratch or improve an existing one. But development may take years. Looking at it realistically, whether there is a good program, a poor program, or none at all, parents still have to face the fact that *it is part of their responsibility to provide some form of education about alcohol at home.* That is asking a lot from parents who are weak on parent/child communication, and it is impossible for parents who have drinking problems (though, interestingly enough, not for many who are recovered alcoholics).

You might profit by obtaining some of the publications used by teachers, most of which suggest ways of developing better communications and showing how teenagers and adults can feel more comfortable discussing a sensitive subject in an objective manner. One way of doing this, for instance, is through what one National Council on Alcoholism (NCA) booklet refers to as "the Spontaneous Interest Approach." * You look for cues in what young people are talking about that provide a natural entry into the subject. For example:

The kids laugh at a sequence on the TV in which a drunk is seen in a humorous incident. Later, you stimulate a family rap session on why the character was funny and actually how close to tragedy humor really is. What would happen if that same drunk had been transferred to a position behind the wheel of a station wagon driving kids and friends home from a picnic?

---

* Peter Finn, "Alcohol. You Can Help Your Kids Cope: A Guide for the Elementary School Teacher," The National Council on Alcoholism, 1977, 12 pages. (Available on request at no charge.)

The subject of poisons and cancer-causing substances comes up, perhaps through a news item about ·dangerous industrial chemicals. You toss out the idea that we ingest a great many chemicals that are harmful without ever paying much attention to the effect on the body—alcohol, for instance. Marijuana has been mentioned earlier several times. Since this is a topic of frequent discussion among teenagers, it could also be a springboard for you to use, if you think you can handle it and not get locked into the subject without ever discussing alcohol. Your leading question might be: "Which is more harmful, pot or alcohol?" The teenagers are more than likely to assert—the climate being what it is today—that marijuana is not really harmful, and certainly less so than hard liquor. Without necessarily endorsing pot, you can easily use this debate to get across some objective information about beer, wine, and liquor. It's a good moment, actually, to come up with the often surprising fact that a can of beer is equal to a glass of wine is equal to a standard cocktail, in alcoholic content and potency.

Beer commercials are an excellent launching point because teenagers are inclined to see right through the hoped-for image of the "macho" beer drinker and make cracks about the advertising. It is easy to start a discussion on the question "Should beer and wine be acceptable for TV commercials? Whiskey is not permitted, yet beer and wine can get a person drunk just as easily, so what is the reason for the regulations?" It doesn't matter whether any conclusions are reached, but only that you lead the talk into a consideration of the nature of alcohol in different forms.

At the dinner table, comments are made about the food at your house versus someone else's. Any discussion of types of foods usually gets into ethnic dishes. From there you can depart into regional and foreign meal habits and the consumption of wine. How do young people feel about drinking wine and why does it cause so many problems in the United States, say, in comparison with Italy, where young children drink wine at the dinner table? (Be careful how you defend family drinking at the table, however; France, where the practice is common, has a high rate of alcoholism.)

A little imagination may be needed to latch on to a commonplace subject and then steer the conversation in the direction of drinking. Don't overdo it and get tagged as a parent who, as one teenager described her father, "doesn't drink much but always seems to have booze on the brain."

As one alcoholism counselor in California, John Vickers, sees it, "Kids who know they are in trouble and are really worried about the situation will talk with almost anyone if it will help lead to a solution. Otherwise, counselors are the ones most likely to establish a good rapport, and the police, probation officers, or other representatives of the law are the least likely."

Parents should participate more in programs designed to encourage dialogues between themselves and their children. Yet they tend to become nervous just thinking about that formidable word, *communications.*

Colleen M. Tinkham, a certified alcoholism counselor for Organism, Inc., in Michigan, has worked extensively with teenagers through dialogues focusing on alcohol and related problems—sometimes over "marathon" weekends. She told me that parents have difficulty with their own feelings (usually fear), especially when their sons or daughters are not of age to be drinking legally. When parents suppress their thoughts and feelings about alcohol use and abuse, instead of being direct and open, they inhibit and delay the process of recovery for the child who has a drinking problem.

What are some common communications blocks?

For research on this book, counselors, teachers, and others in the field of alcohol education were asked questions about communications, rapport, dialogues, and other aspects of adult/youth relationships that affect drinking attitudes and habits. One of the key questions was: "In dealing with young people, from preteens to early twenties, what do you find are the most common communications blocks between parents and children with drinking problems?"

The inability to listen was placed high on the list. When adults decide that it is high time to take some form of action and get through to sons, daughters, or other young people, they limber up their mouths but forget to tune their ears. Teenagers, of course, do the same. They use their voices as the first line of defense, either to excuse what they have been doing or to try to shunt the subject off onto another track. If you have ever attended a successful rap session or heard one that has been taped, you will notice that there is a great deal of listening going on. Certainly, many of the participants are eager to have their say, and a few sometimes hog the floor, but the ears are in gear most of the time, and those in attendance show respect for the opinions of others.

Group rap sessions do have one significant advantage over the kind of one-on-one encounter that takes place when a person initiates a dialogue with a child—they can be more objective and less tense. Even so, *listening* is an effective ingredient.

Denying the problem is an all too frequent block. Tim Hoover of the Pasadena Council on Alcoholism says, "Parents deny that a child has any problem. They assert that 'it's not my kid. He just needs to learn to drink less and stop hanging around those friends!' They protect the kid and take responsibility for any trouble he may get into, which just sends out the message and triggers the reaction 'Hey, this is great. I can continue to drink and if I get into trouble, my parents will take care of me!'"

John Vickers says that when parents adamantly refuse to acknowledge that a son or daughter really has any problem, they will neither face it nor discuss it.

"Another problem is *parents fighting each other*. They do not clearly define a plan of action to help the youth and work against each other. The kid sees this conflict and learns how to manipulate one parent against the other."

Laying down the law almost prohibits communication. Parents who take off on an "authority trip" with the attitude "You listen; I'll talk" stir up plenty of hostility in the child, who would find it difficult to discuss the situation anyway since he is really not aware of the problems he has.

"One of the worst blocks I see," say Hoover, "is when a parent uses the words 'because I said so' or 'because I am your father!' If there is a threatening atmosphere, or the kind of authoritarian behavior that leads to rebellion or feelings of guilt on either side, then a young person finds it impossible to go to his parents and discuss a situation."

"Drinking is a synonym for sinning," commented one young girl. "That's what I was brought up on, religiously and morally. The trouble is, how do you build any kind of dialogue if your parents see only two colors, black and white?"

Gary Olsen, coordinator for a community-based youth counseling program located in a Philadelphia suburb, said, "Parents have a tendency to negate or discount the feelings that their children are experiencing. They may respond with a statement like 'Oh, that's nothing to worry about' or 'It's stupid to be concerned about such a small problem.' This kind of supposed reassurance simply serves to reinforce the interpretation to the child that he or she is bad or wrong, and adds to the confused state of mind."

Sidestepping responsibility causes another block. Attempts at communication between parents and children are wasted time if neither party wants the responsibility for making decisions and resolving problems. As one teenager stated, "I like to sit and rap and listen to people's problems and discuss them. I like getting inside a person and even if it's a bad scene you have a closeness. But I have a real problem with my mother. She wants to talk about things that are good, image-building. The minute I say that I have a problem, she backs off."

On the one hand, the daughter has a good point. On the other, there is sometimes a tendency on the part of young people to try to focus the discussion solely on *parental problems—* whether drinking, money, marital difficulties, or any other negative situation affecting family life. That kind of emphasis also blocks efforts to communicate.

What are some helpful techniques that improve communications?

Adults can often use familiar door openers that young people already understand and will accept. Such approaches were recently explored by a group of boys and girls in their mid-teens at a youth conference in the Blue Ridge Mountains.

"How do we communicate," asked the group leader in opening the discussion, "when it comes to a topic that is as sensitive as drinking, when some or all of the participants have personal problems? If they aren't concerned about their own misuse of booze, then they have to cope with parents or brothers or sisters who are hitting the bottle. It's not easy to talk about such problems."

VERA: If we first say how we feel, that opens the door for others to relate to us. They're feeling nervous and scared, too. When I feel the most scared, then is the time to express the way I feel and I get less scared.

CHERRY: It's like when a girl and boy are having their first date. The boy is scared and so is the girl, and they don't realize how they'll react or what the other person is going through. Sooner or later, they break through the fear and begin talking.

DON: The main standard I have is not to hurt someone else. I can respect another person's opinion even if I don't agree. A lot of kids don't do this. If they know someone has a different opinion, they have to argue it out and try to force their adversary to back down.

Can games have a place in communications?

Games, puzzles, and other devices are tricky. Adults tend to shy away from them because they may seem contrived and tend to stifle communication rather than give it a breath of life. Nevertheless, almost every successful alcohol counselor has developed some games as techniques for getting young people to talk about their problems. A counselor at the Blue Ridge conference said: "I play a little game, but I won't call it a 'device,' because it isn't. It's an exercise, part of limbering up, loosening up, the way an athlete does before a sports event."

In this game, each participant has pencils and paper and the following list of instructions:

1. Name two people with whom you are very close.

2. Describe the place where you have been happiest in your lifetime to date.

3. Describe the place you think you would like to visit most if you had all the time and money necessary to get there.

4. Complete the sentence "Life is a cafeteria where I . . ."

5. List the two facts you would most want a person to know about you, the person being an old friend you have not been in contact with for many years.

6. Now write five words ending in "-ing" that describe you. They don't have to be real words. For example, if you like music you could write "music-ing."

There are, of course, no "good" or "bad" responses. The purpose of the exercise is to get the participants to explore ways of communicating and to understand where some of the hang-ups lie. By discussing which instructions were the easiest or the hardest to comply with, members of the group gain better insights into workable dialogues.

ANDY: I can't complete "Life is a cafeteria. . . ." The problem is that you have not made this clear to me. Are you suggesting that life is made up of a lot of things we have to choose from? Or that we need food, you know, nourishment of all kinds to survive? If we're going to rap, we have to know what we're rapping about.

NELL: You missed the point, I think. Here the whole thing is handed to you on a platter and you just tell what's on your mind. What *you* visualize. Right?

KIRK: The toughest is what two things to tell an old buddy. It's hard to get up there looking down on your whole life—like in a balloon looking down on a city—and pick out what has the most meaning. Sure, you may say it's that you made the football team. But maybe the guy couldn't care less and it's about as much impression as if you said you got a wart on your big toe.

CHERRY: Well, if you know the friend that well, wouldn't you know what she (or if it's a guy) pegs as important in life?

KIRK: Nope. Then you're not rapping for real. You're rapping for what you think someone else wants to hear.

VERA: Would you tell the friend something unpleasant, like you've been hitting the bottle and . . .

DON: No, no. The way I got it here, the way my notes line up, is giving the facts you would *most want* a person to know. Not something that's a disaster.

VERA: So what if you're desperate? You really want this friend to know you've been drinking because if she's a friend she'll maybe help. You say you just won thirty-five dollars in a pool and you're getting across a nothing. Zilch.

LANCE: The easiest way to rap is talking about things like that one point, where you'd like to go if you had plenty of money and time.

NELL: With your parents, you mean? Talking, rapping with adults?

LANCE: Well, anybody. Older, or our age.

DON: I think that's a loaded question. Isn't that an encouragement to escape, *not* to talk about reality but about something you wish would happen, but probably never will?

ANDY: Why don't we go around the room and ask everyone what they would be if they could be anything they wanted? At least that makes us think about what we want to do. It's not totally some kind of trip.

GROUP LEADER: We've gotten to the point here and I think you all have a better understanding of what we mean by communication—reaching through to some other person, or more than one person.

These young people, and others, are of the opinion that the small-group format is excellent and effective and that rap sessions should be short, as well as to the point. If you are trying to encourage a teenager with a drinking problem to seek help through discussion groups, and you have made little headway with other approaches, steer him or her in the direction of programs that are organized around brief meetings with well-defined objectives.

It is perhaps for this reason that more and more teenagers are showing up in Alcoholics Anonymous (A.A.) meetings these days. Sessions seldom last more than two hours. Members speak out explicitly about drinking problems, do not wander into other topics, and show little embarrassment in speaking openly about experiences that can be pretty distasteful. Young people seem to react well to this directness, a kinship with people who can "tell it like it is." Brevity is often refreshing because they are accustomed to detractors, at home, in school, or in the neighborhood, who seem constantly on their backs. They are able to surface in the A.A. milieu, rather than have the feeling that they have been dragged to bottomless depths.

How can parents obtain more help in communicating?

Again and again it has been pointed out by those working with youth problems that the very mention of the word *alcohol* seems to trigger a panic button in parents. Richard Spoonster, director of the Alcohol Education Project at the national office of the Parent-Teacher Association (PTA) in Chicago, called attention to the plethora of "statistics" on drinking that we see in newspapers and magazines, read about in books, hear about over the air. They are shocking, scary, and depressing. Yet their use is often about as meaningful as asserting that if we lined up all the alcoholics in the world, head to foot, they would reach to the moon and back!

What do statistics mean? Some are exaggerated, or apply only to a limited segment of the population. Many are either misinterpreted or just plain false. Sometimes a completely erroneous "statistic" is picked up from a newspaper and spread to other media, although the original editor may be frantically trying to correct a typographical error or point out that the meaning has been changed because the statement was taken out of context.

Parents in one locality were understandably upset by a news headline not long ago: "New Study Reveals that 79% of High School Students in the Region Drink Alcohol." The source for this shocker was cited as a "reliable government study." If readers had the patience to continue to the end (many did not), they would have seen that the headline was completely misleading. What the study had revealed (and this was only a minor aspect of the research) was that by the time they had reached high school, some 79 percent of the students had *tasted* beer, wine, or liquor, but only a much lower percentage could in any way be classed as regular, or even occasional, drinkers.

"No matter what the ages of young people in your family," says Spoonster, "or ones you are directly concerned about, evaluate the situation in proper proportion to the problems—present or anticipated."

One way to avoid panic, to prepare yourself for any crisis, is to think in terms of *prevention*, much as you do in the matter of family illnesses, accidents around the home, or catastrophes on the highway. Alcohol education programs in schools are largely focused on information gathering, personal knowledge, and the prevention of abuse. Most such programs have neither the personnel nor the expertise to commit themselves to corrective action. Nevertheless, rap sessions and other dialogues can often be therapeutic for kids who are having problems.

There are a few programs for parents and other adults scattered around the country, and these are well worth looking into if you can locate one in or near your community. One such program is known as System Training for Effective Parenting (STEP), conducted by Ernest Kennedy, director of the Berkeley County (South Carolina) Commission on Alcohol and Drug Abuse. According to Kennedy and his associate, Helen Clark, "The goal of the program is to create a comfortable home style with open communication between parents and children as a preventive measure against substance abuse."

When the program was first announced, more parents wanted to enroll than could possibly be accommodated. "They approached this with the idea that they could establish a dialogue," explained Kennedy, "if they could get young people to establish better communications. Then they found out that they —the adults—were the ones who needed to lubricate their communications before they could hope for a real dialogue. They began by communicating better with each other and discovered that this was a good step, a necessary step, in communicating with their kids."

What kinds of people participate in prevention programs?

Kennedy emphasizes that most of the participants are "good" parents with "good" families—that is, they are not particularly troubled and do not have histories of problems. Mainly, they want to be informed about alcohol abuse so they can continue to avoid problems. That is why the program is described as "preventive" rather than "corrective."

What do you need to know to be an effective parent? The training kit * and materials for "group dynamics" in the STEP program cover the following subjects:

1. Understanding the behavior, and *mis*behavior, of children. Reasons for the latter, such as trying to attract attention,

---

* Kit available from American Guidance Service, Inc., Publishers Building, Circle Pines, Minnesota 55014, $65. It is valuable as self-help if you cannot locate a program, or for organizing a program.

seeking some form of power or influence, acting in a spirit of revenge.

2. Understanding yourself as a parent. Striving to be a responsible parent, not just a good one.

3. Encouragement. How to build confidence and motivate. Using approaches that are more positive and responsive than the usual kind of praise.

4. Communication. How to *listen* to your children, as well as talk to them.

5. Transmitting your ideas. Learning to be aware of the feelings and reactions of youth. Getting the message across that you are being positive, aware of the needs of youth and the youthful viewpoint.

6. Respecting natural consequences. Letting young people have a voice and the freedom to act on their own.

7. Applying the concept of natural consequences and decision making to other areas of concern.

8. Understanding the value of getting everyone—of all ages—involved. Treating young people like adults in regard to learning, decision making, and the freedom to act.

In the South Carolina STEP program, the kit and materials are not used as lessons in the sense that you might follow a textbook to learn mathematics or chemistry. The topics are presented to the participants as vehicles for motivating the group to open up discussions and get everyone involved.

This kind of open approach is used in many alcohol education programs to develop better communications by giving participants the freedom they need to talk about subjects that are personal in nature and frequently very sensitive.

How do you teach young people to make responsible decisions about drinking?

A youth workshop was held to discuss decision making and responsibility. To kick off the session, the counselor in charge posed this question: An eighteen-year-old boy, living in a state where he is of legal drinking age, plans a party for his teammates at the end of the high school football season. Should he be able to make the decision about serving beer?

BEN: No. It's up to his parents. He's throwing the kegger—if it is one—on his parents' property, isn't he?

MILES: It should be his decision. If his dad has any respect for him, they've already had a dialogue about this kind of situation and the old man has said, "You're old enough to drink, so you're old enough to plan your parties."

MIN: Old enough, but is he experienced enough? or mature enough? So the guy says he's going to have a kegger, not soda pop, but he hasn't had enough experience to think about one point which would be right on his dad's mind: How about some of the younger guys on the team who are not drinking age? Does he serve beer to some, not to others? They all play on the same team, so shouldn't they all have the same refreshments? My vote is that they talk about it and have the father make the final decision.

GROUP LEADER: Okay, but you're really puting the old man on the spot. If he doesn't allow beer to be served to everyone, he gets accused of being a real square. But if he does allow it, he's breaking the law—literally. Mind you, there are no clear-cut answers, no pat formulas for any of these—or say, *most* of these—questions about the suds and sauce. You gotta think 'em through.

Another puzzler: A high school girl is out with her date, who is a college student home on vacation. They're at a cocktail party in a nice home and she (having had only part of one drink) realizes that the guy is getting high. She likes him and doesn't want to be a drag, but how does she handle the problem?

CAROL: That's a toughy because it all depends on one thing—how well can you get through to the date? I've seen this happen to my older sister. If the guy's far enough gone, he won't listen. If he gets argumentative when he drinks, he's going to be obnoxious and probably deliberately gulp more.

RUDY: I know a guy like that—well, several guys who are older —and if they get sloppy and refuse to listen to their date they always feel sorry the next day. And the girl says it's fine to feel sorry now but why didn't you think of that *last night.* So they excuse it by saying, you know, I was a little bombed.

GROUP LEADER: It sounds familiar. There is no real answer, but as Carol suggested, it focuses on whether the girl can get the message across to the guy that she is sober and he is not and she doesn't like the situation. I'd tell any daughter of mine to take a pretty firm stand, make it clear that if her date doesn't shape up she's going to ask around and see who else will take her home—then or later.

Sessions on decision making are vital because they condition young people to think through various situations and help them avoid the pitfalls of being edged into doing things against their will. What it all adds up to, according to Charles E. Dennison, supervisor of an alcohol education program in Minnesota, is that parents must start thinking about orienting their children while they are still youngsters, and not years later when they have come to believe myths and misconceptions and accept a course of action just because "everyone else is doing it."

What should parents do to prevent trouble?

The consensus among young people is that the negative approach—telling sons and daughters not to drink—is *not* the answer. Most kids will drink, or at least experiment. So the most effective strategem parents can employ is to expose children to educational programs that will present the message in a credible manner. Avoid putting alcohol in the tempting category of "forbidden fruit."

Attitudes that regard alcohol use as morally evil tend to be ineffective. "The most effective approach I have found," says Rochester counselor John Zachariah, "is that of educating young people to make responsible decisions. This enables them to choose rationally whether to drink or not to drink." This decision-making process can be facilitated at home by parents and other adults who relate to children during their early developmental stages. "Opportunities must be available to children to participate in the decision-making process in the family and other areas of their life."

In other words, if you have brought up your children to make responsible decisions, you will find it easier to get them to make responsible decisions about alcohol—even though they may appear to be going through a great deal of experimentation with beer, wine, or liquor. If you have not been so fortunate, and you know, or suspect, that a child is having problems with booze, then you are forced into making some of the decisions yourself. This puts you in the position of leading from weakness rather than from strength, but it is no reason for panic.

If your own drinking habits are moderate, then you may be exerting more influence than you realize. Children make unconscious decisions about drinking that are based on what they see in their mothers and fathers. The father who obviously enjoys a glass of beer now and then under pleasurable and relaxed circumstances, and who talks about beer drinking in the same frame of mind in which he might discuss cutting into a tender steak, is getting across a message just as much as though he were to sit down with a son and say, "Look, now, in this matter of teenagers and booze. . . ."

"Adults do make a significant impact on youth," says Zachariah, "although the response to that may be positive or negative. It is important that the adults do not give out conflicting messages and confusing role models through their own drinking behavior."

How do young people develop standards of conduct?

An old Japanese proverb states, "If I give a man a fish, I feed him for a day. If I teach him how to fish, I feed him for a lifetime." A recovering alcoholic aptly applied it to drinking: "If a parent forbids a child to drink at a party, he may keep him sober for one night. But if he teaches him how to respect alcohol, he will keep him sober for a lifetime."

One teenage girl frankly confessed that although she had behaved in a way that was acceptable and comfortable for both herself and her parents where drinking was concerned, she had not actually learned how to make intelligent decisions about alcohol:

TINA: Looking back, I see flaws in my education about the whole matter of drinking. My parents are "average." They face the situation part way, but have to back off because of the gray areas they don't know much about themselves. We had some discussions when I was fifteen and starting to go to high school parties, and I took the stand that I wouldn't drink because it would please my parents if I didn't. They wouldn't have to worry about my getting loaded and looking like a jerk in front of their adult friends. Or worse yet, letting some boy take advantage of me sexually because I was out of control.

Another brief dialogue illustrates a sound parent-child rapport, with guidance toward decision making:

WILMA: I guess I'm what you'd call straight. I talk a lot with my mom, who's great and has always had a lot of fun without getting into trouble. If I'm going to a party, a dance, a dinner date, or any other occasion where there'll be beer, wine, or liquor, I kind of get the signals from her. She'll tell me exactly what she thinks is the right balance for the occasion. It sounds too nicey-nicey, but you know it seems to work. And I have fun.

VIC: How could you have any fun if you're programed like a computer? Suppose you're out with a guy who's going to give you a choice of things to do—dancing or dinner, or a movie, or whatever—do you ask your mother which kind of action is your thing? Or which movie to go to if you pick that?

WILMA: No. Course not. You don't get the point. Those are things I know about and can decide for myself. But drinking is something else. I don't really know yet what it's all about.

Unfortunately, all parents (or guardians) do not approach the problem of drinking in this same spirit, as evidenced by this young man:

TONY: My aunt, who takes care of us, is a religious freak. She can make you feel it's a sin to take a drink. Not wine—that's got some kind of blessing. But she sees you tilting a can of beer and you're a bum. It isn't her saying you're a bum—she makes you feel like one. Guilty!

How do young people help each other to make decisions?

Young people can influence other young people in a positive way, although "peer pressure" is often characterized as a system whereby naughty boys and girls are relentlessly making the rounds trying to get their classmates zonked, so they can have a good laugh, feel superior, or pursue some ulterior motive. It is a fact that abstainers are often referred to with scorn by upper classmen as "squares," sometimes as "fags," in ways intended to puncture their resistance.

By the time children reach high school, particularly as juniors and seniors, personal opinions and outlooks are more respected and pressure is looked upon as a sign of immaturity. Even so, an individual has to exercise a considerable amount of judgment in choosing any particular group or "crowd." In some groups, one may be *expected* to drink, though not pressured. In others, abstention may be the norm.

How much are young people pressured into drinking at parties?

One high school student answered the question this way: "You go to a party and everyone else is holding a beer and you're gonna end up with one, too. Believe me, you're gonna. Just one maybe, you say, but then a second and a third. It's harder for the younger boys and girls, the ones who are impressed at even being invited, or having been able to crash. They feel they're not really 'in' unless they hold a can."

A classmate felt that he had been brought up in the right manner but had never really been educated properly about how to resist pressure when offered a drink. "My aunt and uncle I live with [the mother and father are dead] treated me what I thought was pretty straight. They don't drink much, but they don't get pushy when it comes to telling a kid what to do. They're middle-of-the-road. My problem was I couldn't handle the pressure to have a beer or a drink when my own friends insisted. You could have the best parents in the world, and great communication, and still cave in."

The subject of pressure is explored effectively in a booklet, *Thinking about Drinking,* published by the U.S. Department of Health, Education and Welfare.* Its contents sparked the following discussion among some tenth-grade students in Maryland:

CAROL: The best advice the booklet has is that it gives you suggestions about *not* drinking when you go to a party. I don't mean reasons for not drinking, but how do you *decline* a drink without feeling self-conscious. You say "No thanks," very firmly but in a positive way, and you don't start making excuses for your decision, or apologies, or look embarrassed.

HILARY: It's not always that easy. This boy I go out with is always offering a drink and if I don't take it—maybe only a beer, not necessarily anything stronger—he wants to know why. He's a senior and he knows I'm underage, so it doesn't do any good for me to say that.

CAROL: Say "No thanks." And if he asks why, just change the subject. If he becomes a pest about it, why keep on going out with him?

RUDY: Carol's right. You have to be positive when you answer, and that's that. Not many guys will ask you why you don't take some peanuts if they're passed around and you shake your head. What's so different with a drink? Unless he's trying to get you loaded and, you know—and if that's his game plan, who needs it?

MIN: Let's look at it the other way. Say I'm legal drinking age and having a dinner and all the guests are legal age, too. I'm a good hostess so I offer each person a drink as she or he comes in. I'm not going to ask everybody their reasons why they do or don't take the drink. But also, I have to have some alternatives. And this is a big hang-up at a lot of parties. There's *only* beer, or a very small amount of Coke. You feel silly asking for a glass of water.

MILES: A lot of the time it's because the kids who set up the party are only interested in having a blast. Why fool around with soft drinks?

LINDA: That's not very mature. My mother and father won't let me go to parties like that, not if they know about them.

MILES: You have to be realistic. If you're not exposed to situations like this where you have to make choices, what are you going

* See U. S. Government Printing Office pamphlets listed in Appendix: Further reading.

to do when you're older and on your own and have no parents around to say "No!" to you?

BEN: A person has to take the position that he or she will be okay in a situation where the other guests, as well as the host, are sensible. The guide says that you should *respect* the drinker's decision whether to drink or not to drink. So if you go to one of those blasts where the object is to get as many people smashed as possible, then the element of respect is missing. So you can make your own ground rules and be stubborn about not drinking. Even objectionable.

RUDY: Or repulsive?

BEN: Why not? The people trying to push drinks are being repulsive, so what do you have to lose? On the other hand, if you give in and get loaded, then you're losing two ways—one, because you give in, you let someone else call your signals, and two, because you end up doing just what you were determined not to do—getting bombed.

HILARY: What if I go to this party and I drink but I don't get smashed, loaded, bombed, zonked, or otherwise spaced out?

BEN: Did you go to it intending to have a beer? or a drink?

HILARY: Maybe I didn't really know one way or the other. Does it matter?

BEN: Sure. You've got to rap with yourself ahead of time and say either that you aren't going to drink or you are.

HILARY: What I'm getting at is there's a middle ground. You maybe don't have a choice if your parents have forbidden you to drink and you respect their wishes. But if they give you some ground rules and then . . .

RUDY: How many parents give ground rules? I mean ones we can live with?

HILARY: Mine do, or have been trying to—no liquor, but a little beer is acceptable. So if I go to a kegger and have a beer as a refreshment, that's really in line. If I have the same amount but I drink it to show off or make like I'm a senior, then I'm being stupid.

RUDY: How come your parents *let* you drink beer? You're not old enough.

HILARY: They aren't permissive, if that's what you mean. My dad said that if I went to a party which was under control and I wanted to hold a beer, sip a beer, to be sociable, I could do it. He lets me have a beer once in a while at home. He doesn't go on a crusade about it.

RUDY: Do you think parents should let their kids drink if the parents themselves don't touch the stuff?

HILARY: Sure. Each person has to make a choice on her own.

CAROL: No. Definitely no. If a girl's mom and dad don't drink, she shouldn't either. I mean, later she can, after she's away from home, like having a job or married. But while she's living at home she goes along with the ground rules there. I mean, if her parents serve chicken or hamburgers or stew for meals, no child would think of saying okay but I'm going to eat filet mignon.

RUDY: If parents allow a guy to drink at home, should the guy assume it's a ticket to drinking other places, too?

BEN: He's got to rap with his folks about it and make sure they're talking on the same wavelength. You don't *assume* anything unless you talk it out and agree.

Is it really a good practice to have bars on campus?

By the time teenagers leave home and go off to college, their drinking habits and outlooks are well established. But times change. Let's face it, drinking on campus has become an acceptable practice at many colleges and universities—often a turnaround from the days recalled by the older generations.

Since campuses replace the home when sons and daughters leave the nest to embark on their college careers, it is appropriate to have at least a familiarity with current college attitudes and customs in the matter of drinking. (Not that you can do much about it if your child is already packing his or her bags. But for parents with younger children, it is realistic to look ahead and anticipate the climate.)

The Michigan State program is an excellent example of what can be done to inform students, as well as to assist those who find themselves in trouble because of the bottle, and will be discussed later in this chapter.

Many campuses have their own bars, usually staffed by students. Such bars are not unlike the small pubs you might find in metropolitan areas in almost any section of the United States that is not a "dry" area.

In spite of the fact that alcoholic beverages are thus more accessible than they used to be and that the number of students who drink is higher than it was a generation ago, the problems are no more acute than in localities where there are no on-campus bars. In fact, some administrators find that the problems are less.

"The abuse of alcohol on campus," says T. Alexander Pond,

an officer at the State University of New York at Stony Brook, "is now not nearly as widespread as when I was an under-graduate." Yet Stony Brook has nine bars, six of them run by students, with applications for others pending.

A report from the Rutgers Center of Alcohol Studies also states that college students are not drinking any more (per capita) these days than in the past.

Are students drinking more because alcohol is easily available?

If *availability* were the ingredient leading to problem drinking, the Madison campus of the University of Wisconsin would have drowned in a sea of suds long ago. Beer has been served there since the dormitories were first opened in 1891. Beer, the only alcoholic beverage available on compus, has been served at numerous places, including the Rathskeller and snack bars, where it vies for popularity with soft drinks, coffee, and milk. While most college bars operate on a nonprofit basis, serving drinks at low cost, the Madison campus manages to rack up profits of more than $200,000 a year.

It would be unrealistic to claim that this easy availability is the best way to prevent drinking problems. The University of Wisconsin has had its share of them, and is now making surveys and studying the situation through its Drug Information Center. The important point here is that on campuses all across the country, the subject of drinking is coming more and more into the open and programs are being initiated to counter the prob-lems. It used to be that the very mention of fraternities and sororities conjured up images of beer busts, blasts, and stagger-ing youths. Just to be considered for membership, naive fresh-men and sophomores were more often than not pressured into states of inebriation during the traditional periods of rushing. But that situation is changing, to the great surprise of many an old grad.

Don't fraternities and sororities tend to encourage drinking?

The answer is that campus clubs of any kind can no longer afford to condone heavy drinking, if only for economic reasons—

they cannot pay the cost of repairing damaged property or equipment resulting from drunken escapades. On a higher plane, several national fraternities have become concerned about alcohol abuse and have taken positive steps. One fraternity that has done so is Lambda Chi Alpha, which has more than 10,000 undergraduate members in some 200 chapters in the United States and Canada. "We hope," says Hans G. Reichl, chairman of the fraternity's Alcohol Awareness Task Force and director of residential life at the University of Southern California, "that the program will eventually serve as a model for the entire fraternity world."

The program's first objective is the early identification of members with drinking problems. "When an individual makes a decision to drink, we hope it will be in an intelligent manner," says Executive Director George W. Spasyk. "He ought to know what is safe and what isn't. He ought to know the potential cost of alcohol abuse, to himself and his fraternity."

Spasyk explains that the program is not intended to replace, but to complement existing campus activities designed to combat problem drinking. However, he expressed the opinion that fraternity programs have something of an edge since it is a matter of member helping member, rather than trying to get through to a stranger. Like other campaigns against overindulgence, the Lambda Chi Alpha approach suggests guidelines for members, including these:

- Don't assume it's necessary to serve alcohol at every function.
- Provide alternative, nonalcoholic beverages at parties when alcoholic drinks are available.
- Always offer food when alcohol is served.
- Stop serving alcohol to anyone who gets drunk.
- Close the bar an hour before the scheduled end of the party.

Do college programs offer help to parents in dealing with the drinking problems of young people at home?

One consultant offered this tip for parents who want to get the message across to teenagers, without seeming to be in the position of lecturing: Obtain copies of college publications used in alcohol education programs and use them for family rap sessions or pass-alongs. College alcohol education programs, like the one at Michigan State, put out all kinds of helpful material. Lambda Chi Alpha publishes counsel in fraternity publications, creates posters, distributes a guide, and inserts supplements in its officers' manuals. *

If you are concerned about a high school student who drinks too much and will not pay attention to your opinions, try this ploy: See that he or she has access to some of this college-generated advice about drinking, on a peer-to-peer basis. Maybe that will be more effective than talk. An older sister or brother attending college can also often be more effective than parents in dealing with problems like these.

Other campus Greek-letter organizations are taking action in this arena:

Pi Beta Phi sorority schedules speakers to address members on alcoholism and preventive measures.

Sigma Alpha Epsilon has established a task force to formulate policies on alcohol education and drinking behavior, and the subject is included in its annual leadership school attended by some 500 students and regional officers.

Fraternities and sororities at Ohio State University participate in an alcohol education program, which includes a flyer called *Booze Nooze*. Ohio State has half a dozen pubs and bars on campus, serving beer and wine to students who have reached the legal drinking age.

The Mid-American Interfraternity Council Association, with representatives from several hundred colleges in fifteen states, recently made alcohol the subject of a major session.

The Interfraternity Council of the University of Kansas sponsors "pocket seminars" on alcohol abuse, directed mainly at fraternity and sorority officers in charge of social events.

The University of Florida is developing a program for its fraternities and sororities, which aims at making students more aware of the nature of alcoholic beverages and at establishing guidelines for social conduct on campus and off.

Despite scare headlines about the rise in drinking among

* See Appendix for sources of this kind of information and material.

American youth, adults should focus on those locations, activities, and individuals that are of personal interest and concern. Not every campus is eager to set up bars and spread the good cheer. Harvard University, for example, has only one drinking establishment: Lehman Hall, a cafeteria in Dudley House. It holds a license to dispense beer and wine. But so few students seem to know or care about this local supply of alcoholic beverages that the cafeteria barely sells enough to cover the cost of its liquor license each year.

How does a college alcohol education program function?

Today, most American campuses will offer some form of counsel, if not direct aid, for students having trouble with booze. If you are concerned about a student who seems to be abusing beer, wine, or liquor, you may find unexpected help close at hand. College programs are almost always under the watchful eye of the dean's office, which used to assume the strict role of disciplinarian but fortunately now plays the more amenable and supportive role of counselor.

Like many other colleges and universities, Michigan State University (MSU) had its share of on-campus drinking problems. The legal drinking age in Michigan is twenty-one. But from 1972 until the end of 1978 (when an increase in traffic accidents involving drunken teenagers prompted a reversion), it was eighteen. In order to take a realistic appraisal of the fact that most undergraduates could drink legally, MSU adopted a twofold program in the mid-1970s. It was designed (1) to teach students to drink in a responsible manner and (2) to provide effective assistance for students with serious drinking problems.

Paul M. Oliaro, Director of the Alcohol Education Office, which administered the program, reported that four major resources were helpful in establishing better dialogues between students and staff. The first was a volunteer group from Alcoholics Anonymous, whose members presented information on alcohol abuse in a forthright and knowledgable manner.

"They are widely accepted," he reported, "even by students mistrustful of administration, and we have found them to be . . . our single greatest leverage in changing student attitudes toward drinking."

The second resource was solid training in the techniques of confrontation. Staff members and undergraduate volunteer resident assistants received orientation in proven methods of getting through to students who were alcohol abusers.

The third resource was a publications program, which included the distribution of memos to students, the scheduling of items in undergraduate newsletters dealing with alcohol desensitization, and requests for playbacks of opinions on various aspects of alcohol abuse.

The fourth resource fell into the legal category, making staff members and students aware of laws and regulations for which they would be held responsible in the matter of alcohol consumption and property damage, disturbances, or casualties related to drinking.

The university's policies were geared to reflect this realistic approach to living with alcohol, and were in fact used as models for programs by other colleges—some in areas where the drinking age is still eighteen or nineteen. One significant ruling was that at least 25 percent of the beverages offered at social events be *non*alcoholic. "This policy," reported one member of the staff, "resulted in a decrease in the misuse of alcohol and increased attendance at such events by those who chose not to consume alcohol."

How do you approach a young adult with a drinking problem?

The undergraduate volunteers working the Michigan State program found that in order to be effective they had to be able to look at themselves and understand their *own* attitudes and behaviors in the matter of alcoholic beverages, drinking, and the handling of problems. Indeed, the values that are essential in establishing rapport with young people are those that each of us holds as truths about ourselves and about the world around us. Many times we find that each of us has one set of values for ourselves and another set for others.

Bonnie G. Olson, coordinator of MSU's alcohol education program, passed along a checklist entitled "Basic Confrontation Techniques." It has been refined and perfected over several years in this program of "people helping people."

The techniques are well worth studying by parents, teachers, counselors, and other interested adults because they are particularly realistic and effective in establishing a dialogue.

- Be simple and direct as you speak, but proceed openly and smoothly. *Rushed* encounters are self-defeating.
- Know the facts, as well as you can, but do not try to come across as an "expert."
- Be specific. You are zeroing in on the person's *drinking* behavior, not general behaviors and attitudes. (If a boy has made a mess of his room because he got drunk on beer, don't get into a discussion of his generally sloppy habits.)
- *Care!* At every opportunity, communicate your real interest in the young person—whether as parent, relative, teacher, or friend.
- Don't be afraid to show your feelings (anger, for example), yet make sure that they are directed at the *behavior*, not the person.
- Try to make the confrontation *objective*, in terms of the behavior. You can be subjective, though, when it comes to your relationship to the person.
- Stick to the issue—the problem is drinking. Don't let yourself be led into unrelated or marginal subjects.
- Avoid any "I told you so!" inferences.
- While the person is still inebriated, do not use arguments or threats to try to make your point. Wait until later to make the confrontation, when the person is sober.
- Be prepared for excuses, promises of change, accusations that *you* drink (or have other behavior problems), assertions that this is "no big deal," and attempts to switch the subject.

11 | Why do young adults need to know more about alcohol?

Things are changing. Today, young people are calling the signals more and more.

Look around you and you will see evidence that changes are taking place because of what young people—not their parents or older relatives—have decided to do, or not do. Attitudes toward education, marriage, living together, careers, women's rights, religion, communication, and life-styles are vastly different from those commonly held a generation ago.

The same can be said about the use of alcohol.

Traditionally, four areas have held the key to teenage drinking, according to the Education Commission of the States: the home, the church, the school, and the law. In recent years a fifth area, *the peer group,* has come to exert strong influence. No longer is it effective to set down rules which must be obeyed. Nor do the youth of today give uncritical acceptance to statements by teachers, parents, or other adults.

Dr. Gail Gleason Milgram, director of education at the Center of Alcohol Studies at Rutgers University, New Brunswick, New Jersey, points out that adults tend to overlook the real meaning of adolescence. "Often this period is considered only a preparation for life," she says, "when actually it is a time of accomplishment and satisfactions as well as preparation and experimentation. If teenagers are viewed as active decision makers in the educational process, it becomes clear that decisions and opinions regarding alcohol use are experimented with and formulated during adolescence."

Why, then, does the issue of teenage drinking cause so much alarm? If you will reflect on American history, you will recall that the drinking of alcoholic beverages has sparked controversy, even major social upheavals, down through the generations. Deep-rooted feelings on the issue, made more acute by the years of Prohibition and the battles for Repeal, have not really been shaken off, despite assertions that we live in a more sophisticated and enlightened age.

"Though alcohol use is a socially accepted custom in the United States today," says Dr. Milgram, "substantial disagreement and uncertainty remain regarding drinking customs and alcohol use."

One strong reason why we panic when faced with teenage drinking problems, real or imagined, is that our information is likely to be sparse, sprinkled with myths, and often biased. Many adults could not pass a simple true-false test on the nature of alcohol and the effects of alcoholism. We see the subject in the form of scare headlines and unsettling national statistics.

"Teenage drinking is usually presented by the mass media," says Dr. Milgram, "as a significant problem causing death-by-auto, pregnancy, and antisocial acts. It is also presented as an area to be concerned with but avoided, as there is no consensus as to whether or how teenagers should be taught to drink or prepared to live in a drinking society."

Dr. Milgram reports that the majority of teenagers drink alcoholic beverages and that by the age of nineteen, "the proportion of teenage users of alcohol closely mirrors the proportion of adult users," which is approximately two thirds of the population. Young people did not create for themselves this world of social drinking—they simply entered into it as part of an existing environment. It is all the more important, then, that they should learn what this environment consists of—about alcohol in general and about specific types of drinks in particular. "They need to know how it should be used," says the booklet distributed by the Education Commission of the States, "and how it should not be used. They need to know why abuse of alcohol can result in unplanned difficulties, and how its proper use, by those who choose to drink, can serve a useful social function."

What do we mean by "problem" drinking?

A counselor tried to clarify this question by asking members of a workshop group what they thought the term implied, with the following results:

RALPH: By "problem drinker," you mean maybe kids who go out for lunch and drink beer?

GROUP LEADER: Could be, but certainly the ones who do and always let themselves get out of control. Or who sneak drinks between periods and arrive in classrooms feeling high, maybe strung out, and then getting the teacher and other students on edge.

GARY: A lot of young people say okay, I drink but it's my own thing and I'm the one who has to live with the flak. Is that realistic? Every problem drinker affects three or four other people adversely—all the way from just being a nuisance to committing violent acts.

GROUP LEADER: Suppose a boy goes into the bathroom at his home and lifts the top of the toilet tank and takes out a bottle and drinks straight from the neck. Would you think he was a little nuts?

BETH: Could it be because his parents forbid liquor in the house?

GROUP LEADER: This is not normal behavior, no matter what the excuse. An alcoholic may hide bottles in the toilet tank, the air conditioner, and any place else they could fit. Sometimes he may not recall where he has all his bottles stashed away. But some drinkers are very ingenious at finding places to stash away their supplies. Drink is the focus of all of their energies.

Some young newcomers to A.A. in New Haven, Connecticut, described typical problems:

JULIA: I got so messed up that I came here as a last resort. Frankly, I expected to find a room full of zombies. I don't know how I took so many jolts and got so hungover so often without any adults ever catching on. I was sent away to school because I was failing four of my five subjects. My mother thought I was under too much pressure. My father didn't have any opinion except that I ought to get a fresh start. They never suspected I had liquor stashed away all over the place. My "fresh start" took the form of finding hiding places around the school where upper-class monitors and the teachers wouldn't think of looking for booze. I was brown-bagging it all over. Always stoned. But I was clever now at hiding the fact . . .

ERNIE: Before I came to my first A.A. meeting, my sponsor said to me, "Look, Pigeon, here's something I want you to read and memorize. If you don't do one other goddam thing." He gave me the serenity prayer: "God grant me the serenity to accept the things I cannot change, courage to change the things I can, and wisdom to know the difference." He had me pegged from the first countdown. I was always trying to change things that couldn't be changed, and using the bottle to do it. I didn't have the guts to try to change the things I could—like my drinking. And I sure didn't know the difference about anything. To play it safe, I kept pretty well spaced out and never rapped with adults or squares my own age—only the other lushes.

GUS: I smashed up the car several weeks ago. I was half-bombed. But that wasn't the reason I ran off the road and into an abutment—although the police and my parents thought so, and still think so. What I really was doing was trying to commit suicide. I had tried it once before, with pills and booze. I threw up before a lethal enough dose got to me and was in the horrors for two days. Nobody ever knew, not until right now when I told you. It's all from the booze. It messes up my brain and if I can't seem to self-destruct, I better find out how to get off the sauce and sober up.

BUNNY: My mother would kill me (my father's dead and my stepfather is always away) if she knew I came to A.A. I tried to tell her one time I thought I was having a drinking problem, which my real father had. But she gave this nervous laugh she has and said I was exaggerating. A friend of hers said she was trying to get her husband to go to A.A. and Mom blew up and called A.A.-ers bums, hookers, and deadbeats.

IRENE: I'm here because I'm scared. Scared at what it's been doing to me lately when I have any drinks. And I can't remember what I did. My girl friend told me the other day that I'm off her list because I took off my clothes and tried to seduce her boyfriend. I didn't have any idea what she was talking about. And one guy in our class was making crude jokes and saying I had been, you know, intimate with him after a party. How could this be, since I hate the guy anyway? But I really don't know. Am I really losing my memory? What can I do about all this?

RODNEY: I drove thirty miles to come to this A.A. meeting because I need help, but I don't want anyone in my hometown to see me and think I'm a drunk. A permanent drunk, not just having an occasional blast. I can't do anything anymore without sneaking some drinks first. If I go out with a date, I need a drink first. If I have an exam coming up, I tilt a bottle a couple of times before going into the exam. I can't sleep now unless I have a couple of beers. Or a brandy. I hope this is the right place to come to because my problem gets worse and worse, and if my old man knows what's going on he'll. . . .

HOPE: My parents don't drink. It's our religious belief. They threw my oldest brother out of the house two years ago because he was drinking beer and wine. They don't know about me, but I started drinking wine at friends' houses and now I can't stop. Not for more than a few days. I'm frightened to think what my father will do when he finds out. And how can he *not* find out, sooner or later?

What are some social consequences of problem drinking?

Young people who end up as tragic statistics very often had little or no alcohol education and are not in the least prepared to cope with the potent and dangerous drug, alcohol. Why is it that our schools more often than not fail to provide adequate alcohol education?

"I went to my ten-year reunion a while back," said Gary Fair, "and it was easy to observe that many of the classmates who were in trouble—divorced, with jail records, losing jobs, or bombed at the reunion—started to have drinking problems while they were still in school."

College administrators find there is a high correlation between the consumption of alcohol on campus and the incidence of brawls, noise, disruptive behavior, and property damage. Vandalism is a major area of crime for youngsters in their early and midteens who have been drinking. You have undoubtedly been outraged many times over at the sight of, or reporting of, such acts of wanton destruction. They range from obscene graffiti on the walls of schools and other public buildings to smashed windows, ripped-out plumbing, and arson. "Time and again," said an editorial in the March, 1978, *Kiwanis Magazine* report on vandalism, "drug and alcohol abuse are related to vandalism." Joseph Keglovits, a Bethlehem, Pennsylvania, crime prevention officer, points out that alcohol gives youths a false sense of courage, and under its influence, they will do things they wouldn't ordinarily do.

"A chilling example of this occurred in Bellevue, Washington, an affluent suburb of Seattle. A group of youths were drinking beer near the high school's learning resource center. After many cans had been consumed, one of the teenagers suggested that they burn the school. They set fire to the building, causing a $1 million loss of facilities, books, and audiovisual materials."

About half of all homicides are caused by drinking. You have to consider, too, the enormous tax burden when public funds must be diverted to fighting alcoholism and the destructiveness caused by drinkers.

"Every juvenile I know who has been an offender," reports Fair, "either drank too much or had an alcoholic parent."

Why does a teenager drink to the point where it leads to infractions of the law and later to serious juvenile delinquency? If a fifteen-year-old boy seems to be attending only those parties where alcohol is served, the drinking problems that ensue may be a camouflage for underdeveloped social skills. A fourteen-year-old who drinks may be using beer or wine to hide feelings of anxiety related to situations where he feels uncomfortable even with his peers. "Alcohol temporarily dulls this discomfort," says New Jersey police psychologist Elva Herzog, "and imparts an artificial feeling of control to the youngster. However, if the learning of social skills is bypassed at this point in life, later the child will be faced with a serious deficit in social skills and the chance of being socially handicapped."

What do you do when a young drinker is in trouble with the law?

The first consideration is not so much educating the child, but *orienting the adult.* "If a youngster under the legal drinking age has had police involvement stemming from the use or misuse of alcohol," explains Herzog, "the adult talking with the youngster must first be aware of the youngster's initial attitude toward the incident, which will be denial and resistance to an examination of his or her behavior."

As she sees it, the young offender is immediately placed in a defensive position because acknowledgment of drinking (underage) is automatically an admission of guilt and wrongdoing. For an adult to ask a young person to admit to breaking the law is often a futile endeavor. Yet that is precisely what most adults will do, under the mistaken impression that this is a necessary step in resolving the situation. "This approach to conversation will only force most youngsters to deny facts, lead to accusations and further denials, and thereby block effective communication."

How should you handle it?

Simply accept it as fact that the child has been drinking,

without making accusations or threats, and proceed from that point. "When parents talk with their children about drinking," she advises, "they should be knowledgable about their own feelings and fears. Are they afraid that the child is becoming another link in a family chain of alcoholism? Are they fearful that this is another demonstration of independence by a child, a fact that they are already having difficulty accepting?"

Can problem drinkers always get help?

HECKY: I've had a couple of drinks. But I was on the wagon. For ninety days I was—ninety days means something like a lifetime to me. I never gave up the booze that long since I started drinking at about age thirteen, six years ago.

For me, drinking is bing, bing, bing, *bing*! I mean, it's a subway train. It's a lot of cars tied together—glasses of booze, not cars. And it bounces along inside me, too. I could hit my head, bash my head, sprawl on the floor, hug the center pole, and try to keep from the dizzies. But it would be all along the subway train. Rumbling, noisy. Each one maybe like having square wheels. You know what I mean? Not unless you've been there yourself, with the glasses strung out, the bottle. Getting bombed.

I worked on a subway last summer. I hung on between the cars and told people to get the hell away from the edge of the platform. I broke up fights, a couple with knifers. Would I have done it not having a drink? You'd have to be crazy to think so. When someone's ugly and flashing steel, you don't hang around if you're sober. You know what steel does to you? No pain any more than a little razor nick you get shaving. But wow! Your flesh all opened up like the way you tear open an envelope.

The subway, it's one hellhole job. I did lots of better jobs, nothing jobs. In the freight yards. Truck driving. Bartending. Painting bridges. Collecting garbage—and stray cats and dogs—and deadbeats for an agency. They all thought I was older because I always had an I.D. card, faked to over twenty-one so I could get booze anytime, anywhere.

Hecky has been up and down, drunk countless times, in his young career as an alcoholic. He has been in A.A. for only short periods, although periodically he gets what he describes as a compulsion to go.

A guy has to *talk* to other people once in a while. Sure, I talk in bars to the bartender or strangers. I talk on the job with other workers, mostly while we're popping a six-pack. I talk to myself when I'm bombed, maybe looking in the mirror and telling myself what a jerk I am.

But that's not *talking*. Not like when a kid is rapping with his old man or maybe some other adult who is really listening, not just sitting there and nodding and putting you on. The nearest I've come to any kind of dialogue has been in A.A. I got pride. You wouldn't think so, me being not always in the best of shape. But in A.A. the group treats you like you're a person. You can level with them. No one gets insulted or annoyed or gives you the idea you don't really know anything. Even the old-timers, the ones who've been in the program twelve or fifteen years and know you're only a pigeon will say, "Okay, Hecky, you have an opinion to express. You say it like you feel it, not like you think *we* want to hear it. And if we got any complaints or bitches, we'll say it like it is, too.

Dennis is struggling to rehabilitate himself. An alcoholic, age thirty, he has been in trouble with the law about two thirds of his life, largely because of booze, but he is recovering. He has a story to tell, although for a long time his lips were sealed because he was in prison, serving fifteen years for having robbed a liquor store.

"We do not permit prisoners to be interviewed," explained the counselor on the warden's staff who assists in the rehabilitation of inmates with alcohol- and drug-related problems. "Too many criminals have been exploited for purely mercenary reasons and without much benefit, if any, to the individuals in our charge."

Dennis feels strongly that he has to try to get his message through to the world beyond the bars, and I was finally allowed to question him. Here is his story, based on his brief answers:

Dennis had his first drink when he was nine and was drinking "a lot" by the time he was eleven. Because of his need for booze, money was a huge problem. "I wasn't able to make any money, but I needed it. So that led to the other problem at the same time—trouble with the cops." He began stealing, and his first brush with the police came at the age of eleven.

I wanted a drink and didn't have any, so I broke into a bar and liquor store. I was with another kid. I never did anything by myself in those days. Sometimes we'd find a guy who'd buy liquor for us, but this time we couldn't find any guy who wanted to make a buck or liked to see little kids get smashed, so we thought, why not just take it?

All we wanted was to get high. Nothing else seemed to matter to us but the fun we would have later on. If it wasn't for the kicks, the fun, we wouldn't have broken into the place.

Dennis and his friends were not drinking beer or wine, but "hard stuff."

The stronger the better. My buddies and I used to chug-a-lug it, to see who could drink the most booze at one time. Did we like the taste? No, I hated the taste. But I knew to get high I had to drink it hard. We never drank beer because you had to put away a lot of it to get any kicks. And you couldn't lug around a lot of six-packs on foot.

When I asked Dennis if he recalled any _good_ experiences he had with drinking, he said:

That's funny! You know, the good times, if there ever were any, I can't remember. But the _bad_ times—they're clear as day. And a lot of them. . . !

Everything was a joke, at first. We had fun, no matter what we did when we were drinking. But I can't remember just what kind of fun. Getting sick, though, and puking, and breaking into places, I do remember. And passing out. I remember times coming to in strange places, like the woods. . . .

The more I drank, the less I cared about anything. And the funnier everything became to me . . . well, screwier, nuttier, not with it.

He fully realized and admitted that booze was the cause of his being in prison.

If you think of it in the way I ripped off the liquor store because I needed booze, because I was in such bad shape that it didn't matter to me what I did to get some drinks. Actually, it was more because I had been drinking than needing it. There's no such thing for me as "plenty."

Did he recall the arrest that led to his long prison sentence?

It was at night and I had been drinking and I kept thinking that tomorrow would come and what was I going to do then. I thought most of the night about hanging it up, but something happened to me, inside. The more I drank, the madder I got because I didn't have the courage to hang it up, to kill myself. And the madder I got, the more I drank. I have to tell you that I never did like to get bombed. I always wanted to get high, and stay there. But that particular night I really got smashed and somehow was going to change things by robbing a liquor store.

This clerk in the liquor store, he made me even madder when I went in, as if he was the one who had gotten me drunk. I had an urge to take everything out on him. After I held him up, I felt good. I really did. It was like a big joke. The money didn't really matter that much to me after all.

Dennis had been arrested many times before that, "all from booze in one way or another. Breaking in, drunk and disorderly, fights, stealing, resisting arrest."

I asked him if he thought he might have achieved sobriety if he had ever had some help.

Many, many times I did have help, but I could not stop drinking and getting into trouble. I had the *best* help you could get. When I knew it was impossible for me to stop, then I tried to kill myself. Two times I OD'd on "tranks," but came out of the coma in a hospital. I didn't want to live, and I couldn't make it to the cemetery either. That's tough!

Dennis told me several times that he hoped his case could be presented because it might help young people to understand more about the disabling power of alcohol when used by kids who are too young to realize the dangers. For teenagers who are starting to have drinking problems, Dennis advised:

Tell them to get into some *counseling*, where they have people *to talk to.* When I was a kid, drinking was way out because there was *no one* I could talk to, or turn to. Self-help programs are the best, where kids can talk with others but still be able to take responsibility, to make some decisions.

He also added that if parents want to get through to kids about drinking they have to start early in life.

You have to start early. Essentially that means with *love*. There are many ways, but love is one of the very biggest and best. And *caring*. I could never talk to my own parents. The love just wasn't there, or the caring. If adults would just look around them, they would see that this was true.

Communicating is everything.

Parents who are confused about what to do when a child has a drinking problem can often get valuable counsel by speaking informally with young people who themselves have been in trouble but are recovering.

Gary Fair zeroed in on the following tips to parents who know, or suspect, a child is using alcohol or drugs:

• Don't panic. Many young people experiment with alcohol and drugs and never get into serious trouble.

• If a problem does exist, preaching is a waste of time.

• Be honest and open and try to find out the extent of involvement, at the same being prepared for denial and rejection.

• Be patient and caring.

• Be an active listener, then deal first with whatever problems the child is willing to talk about.

• Do *not* try to solve their problems for them or make decisions for them because if you do the problems are going to get worse, not better.

What do you do in an emergency?

You may not know how to locate a person you can talk with in an emergency situation, one who is qualified to give advice, through either personal experience or professional training. But there is almost always someone just a phone call away— at the other end of a "hot line." This is simply an emergency telephone number that people in need of help can call at any hour of the day or night.

"Hot line! Can I help you?"

Those or similar words will be the first ones you hear after you dial the number. The speaker will probably be one of several hundred carefully screened volunteers who have been trained to provide instant assistance, and to advise the caller how to obtain further help. You do not have to identify yourself or anyone concerned, or reveal the neighborhood in which you live. In fact, the only information you have to disclose is the nature of your problem and the kind of help you are seeking.

Most large cities have hot lines to cover a variety of crises, and even smaller cities and towns are establishing such services. They may be called "dial-for-help" services, "lifelines," or "listening posts." If you can't find one, ask the operator for help, or call any number listed under "A.A." or "Alcoholics Anonymous."

12 | *What are adults doing about the overall problem?*

Many of the activities to counteract drinking problems among youth go on behind the scenes, and receive very little publicity. But the subject is coming more and more out in the open. Canada has pioneered a program that has attracted considerable attention and could serve as a model for other locations. Perhaps parents can learn something about encouraging communications with their children from a brief look at how Canada's Department of Health and Welfare focuses on the problem with a series of advertisements entitled "Dialogue on Drinking." One headline reads:

Drinking. If we don't talk about the problem, we'll never start to solve it.

"Talking about the problem is not an answer, but it's a start," states the text.

Talk to the guy across the street, to your teenagers about drinking habits. Tell your friends when you think they've had enough to drink. If you speak in support of responsible use, you will encourage others to do the same as you do—if you are responsible.

More than 2,000 responses to the first ad inspired the second:

Now you're talking . . . !
You are talking about some of the problems and that brings them into the open.

Suggestions quickly and steadily came in advocating in-school educative programs, a radio or TV series that would show *realistically* what happens when a person drinks too much, and courses for teenage girls who are intent on marrying young, to advise them on handling drinking situations and inebriated husbands.

Action, as well as talk, was documented as one of the results of the campaign. "In Ontario, the Thunder Bay Committee for Dialogue on Drinking is well on its way. . . . In St. Catherine's, Ontario, the Parent Communications Program is dealing with alcohol and other problems. . . . In Rothesay, New Brunswick, forty Knights of Columbus have asked how they can help. Medicine Hat, Alberta, has its Alcohol in the Community program. . . . And in Vancouver, teenagers petitioned against opening two liquor stores because some of their friends had been killed by drunk drivers."

One correspondent reported, "I see my own peers' attitudes changing. Instead of bragging how drunk we got on a particular night, we are more apt to take pride in being able to control our consumption to a reasonable level."

How does a community program work?

The Yak Shack	The Way Up
Ziggy's Place	The Place
The Open Door	Aquarius

What are these—bars? titles of new television shows? quaint restaurants? No, they are the names created for "rap rooms" that are located in all of the junior and senior high schools in Florida's Dade County. These are places where kids can drop in any time, talk about their hang-ups, socialize, or get the ear of an ever-present counselor who is adept at the art of listening. The students themselves are the ones who have designed, decorated, named, and sometimes equipped the rap rooms.

"When do we use Ziggy's?" echoed one teenager, speaking in effect for all rap rooms in the whole county. "Whenever we like. We drop in for one-on-one raps, or with groups. We may have a scheduled session, but informal. Or a class, more formal.

Some kids are there all the time, and others only when they feel low or out of it."

Rap rooms make up only one facet of the Professional Resources in Developmental Education program, known as PRIDE. Other aspects and activities include parent communication, value clarification, decision making, student counseling, teacher training, community action, alcohol and drug education, rehabilitation programs, health improvement, and even music, yoga, and the development of creative crafts.

PRIDE is directed at:

Students. "Have a problem, or willing to help someone unravel his? Enjoy working with younger students? Contact the PRIDE resource specialist in your school and find out how you can get involved."

Parents. "Are your lines of communication open? Feel fenced out of today's youth scene? Call the PRIDE resource specialist at your school, just to talk if you wish."

Teachers. "Do you know about your school's PRIDE program? Learn more about how it can assist and affect you. . . ."

You do not live in Dade County or even in Florida? The program sounds excellent and badly needed, but is too remote from your community and your problems? Your community might well be able to benefit from what Dade County has learned, no matter how far away you may be. Don Samuels, Coordinator of the PRIDE program, invites inquiries. Write him at: Dade County Public Schools, Suite 309, 1444 Biscayne Boulevard, Miami, FL 33132.

PRIDE is not limited to alcohol- and drug-related problems and education. But it is especially effective in this area because the program brings together all of the types of resources that are necessary to help young people: education, counseling, discussions, communication, and involvement, to name a few. Of great importance, as has been noted with a number of other community programs discussed in this book, one of the basic activities is peer counseling. More than 5,000 peer counselors have been trained in the techniques of active listening, clarification of values, and decision making. Peer counselors have worked with more than 20,000 students in group situations and hundreds of others in individual exchanges, helping them to resolve their own hang-ups and hassles.

"We feel that personal pride begins early in life," says Samuels, "so the PRIDE program follows the same principle. By use of what we call our "Magic Circle," at the elementary level, youngsters get to experience group discussions, express themselves, and discover that others may or may not feel the way they do—but that's okay. They learn to give and take, and in the process, *be someone.*

"With this kind of start, the program involves the kids as they grow older—and not only the kids but parents, teachers, and the whole community."

Should we focus only on drunkenness?

A report from the Addiction Research Foundation (33 Russell Street, Toronto, Ontario, Canada M532 S1) emphasizes a viewpoint that is sometimes overlooked:

We have often failed to recognize the fact that the majority of young people who choose to drink do not end up dead, or in hospital, in jail, or pregnant. We usually fail to acknowledge that there are distinct pleasures and real benefits in drinking alcoholic beverages in an appropriate and nondamaging way. This one-sided, negative kind of teaching, which runs contrary to the experience of a great many young people . . . substantially reduces the believability of all our teaching.

Parents and other adults lose their credibility with the young when they, consciously or not, adopt this negative viewpoint. And far too many programs do, since alcohol education owes its very birth in part to temperance movements. Overemphasizing abstinence and focusing on the tragic results and dire consequences of drinking generates the undesirable idea that getting loaded, smashed, zonked, or stoned is the *normal* condition of those who drink. Drinking in moderation and still remaining sober is a situation that fades away into oblivion and is not even considered possible.

Adults too often fall into the trap of tagging a bender, brawl, or blast as evidence of alcoholism. Deplorable though such misconduct may be, it is not necessarily a sign that all participants are alcoholics, or even budding alcoholics. A recent editorial in *The Journal of Alcohol and Drug Addiction,* on drinking behavior, warns, "To overreact to an individual's experimentation or use [of alcohol] by labeling him an alcoholic, an addict, or other similar term may result in a lowered self-concept and, particularly if this labeling is public, may result in social exclusion. To lower another's self-concept is particularly undesirable in that a favorable self-concept tends to serve as a deterrent to deviant behavior."

Should we ignore the pleasurable side of drinking?

A more positive viewpoint was expressed in *Health Education* in an article entitled "Alcohol Education and the Pleasures of Drinking." The author, Peter Finn, a senior education and training analyst in Cambridge, Massachusetts, deplores the fact that most educational materials published for use by teachers and students "fail to communicate adequately the significant ways in which alcohol gives pleasure," and, in fact, "focus overwhelmingly on the dangers of alcohol abuse."

Why should we not, asks Finn, explore the rationale for stressing some of the pleasures and comforts of drinking? Most young people know that the average American finds drinking a pleasurable experience. "As a result," says Finn, "when educators fail to discuss this enjoyment at some length, they risk losing a student's confidence in the trustworthiness of what they have to say about alcohol *abuse.*"

We can hardly carry on any kind of dialogue with our young people if we ask them to close their eyes to the realities. They are aware that:

- For many families, wine is as much a part of dinner as soup or bread or dessert.
- Countless numbers of drinkers enjoy a cold glass of beer to quench the thirst on a very hot day.
- Extra flavor and tenderness can be brought out of meat, fish, or fowl by cooking it in wine.
- Flavoring desserts with liqueurs can add a touch of elegance, as well as improved taste.

• Collecting and sampling fine wines can be a fascinating and even rewarding hobby.

• Wine has played a vital part in religious observances for thousands of years and in some instances is all but obligatory.

• In some instances, alcoholic beverages are used for medicinal purposes, on the advice of doctors and others in the field of health.

A school alcohol education program that realistically and objectively discusses the beneficial aspects of drinking, says Finn, has established the credibility necessary to move into a discussion of the dangers and abuses. "Alcohol education must begin to face the challenge of presenting alcohol use and abuse in a balanced framework," he cautions, "which does not obscure the pervasive reality of responsible and enjoyable drinking in America."

The comment applies equally well to any parent or other adult who intends to discuss drinking problems with a young person and wants to minimize that old bugaboo, the credibility gap.

With whom do young people have the best rapport?

Parents frequently are puzzled by the difficulties they seem to encounter trying to get through to their kids, while the kids seem to have no trouble talking with their peers, some of the teachers, or other adults. Counselors involved with alcohol education programs were asked the following question: "Many dialogues, from informal rap sessions to more structured discussions, seem to break the ice jam. With which groups do kids in trouble seem to have the best rapport: their peers, parents, teachers, counselors, doctors, ministers, law-enforcement officials, or others?"

Tim Hoover, who started drinking at the age of fifteen and experienced serious difficulties in school, with the law, and in his young adult life before finding his way to recovery and eventual involvement as an alcohol counselor, is in a good position to reflect on this.

"I see that peer influence is the greatest factor in the use of people," he says, "young or old. I think that young people who have been through the hell and have found their way out of the hell, have the greatest influence. I do see, though, that no matter who you are, if you approach young people with a nonmoralistic, nonjudgmental attitude, and let them know that the ultimate decision is theirs, not yours, then you can break through the jam. Compassion and the willingness to *listen* are great prerequisites in dealing with young people who may be in trouble."

David Huberty, the Central Minnesota detoxification counselor, feels that kids in trouble "have the most frequent, yet perhaps the most superficial, rapport with their peers. They frequently have the poorest rapport with those persons with whom they really need the best rapport—their parents." Eventually, the person who manages to get through to them most effectively is likely to be neither a peer nor a parent but rather some other adult figure who has shown genuine interest and has to some degree taken a risk in confronting the youth about his inappropriate behavior and problems. At the same time, though, that adult is the one who communicates a general acceptance of the young person in trouble and holds out realistic hope that there can be improvement.

Looking back on his experience, Kansas City counselor Gary Olsen says that kids may appear to be suspicious of everyone but themselves and their own age group, yet they really will listen to the words of an adult at times. "Peer groups, with counselors present to keep the participants focused on the subject, seem to achieve the greatest rapport," he reports. "The worst rapport is probably with law-enforcement officials. But these are generalizations and I am not too comfortable with pronouncing such opinions unless I know more of the specifics—the problems and individuals involved."

His comments, however, are backed up by other counselors, including Eddie McNees of Tennessee, who is of the opinion that "kids in trouble seem to have the best rapport with their peers and the worst rapport with law officials." If it is any consolation to you, parents seem to stand somewhere in the middle, and the ones who approach this sensitive area with an open mind, and after having done their homework on the nature of alcohol and alcoholism, are likely to manage quite well.

What can parents learn from peer education programs?

Parents often find they cannot bridge the communication gap or exert a healthy influence on their children in situations where alcohol is a major part of the problem. Says Joanne Trejo, program director of the Teenage Alcohol Program (TAP) in Van Nuys, California, "Dialogue is probably more inhibited than with other kinds of problems. Many factors complicate communications, such as the parents' attitudes and prejudices about drinking, or denial on the part of a young person that he has been abusing alcohol."

TAP, a voluntary organization, is described as "neither wet nor dry." It does not attempt to turn young people into abstainers. Rather, its primary goal is to eliminate the social stigma attached to alcoholism through public education. It provides information and referral services for the general public, and develops suitable resources and services in the region. TAP has become known, for example, as a place where young people can go to talk privately about problems, whether their own or those of friends or relatives. Alcohol education classes are offered on a ten-week basis, with schedules of rap sessions, speakers, films, and group projects. Many youthful drinkers have recovered because they have been able to talk with their peers through programs such as that offered by TAP.

"Past experience has proven to me," says Trejo, "that peers or someone close to the age of the young person in trouble, who has experienced similar problems and can speak the same language, will be most effective." Young people are also inclined to listen to an adult who has "been there," as in the case of TAP in Antelope Valley, California. Director John Vickers has been successful through "eyeball-to-eyeball" contact almost daily with teens whose boozing has gotten them into serious trouble. He is himself a recovered alcoholic.

This viewpoint is shared by Terry Royer, a health education consultant with the county alcohol control program in Riverside, California. "I have developed a successful program for high school students called Peer Education Resource Training, where individual students are taught how to do peer education and cross-age teaching. The response in the schools and in the community has been very positive."

He works not only with teenagers, but with children as young as nine or ten. "It's a whole new ball game," he commented. "We never used to think of kids that young as having such problems, but now we know they do."

Can young people help each other?

Royer starts a program by first working with parents and teachers, forming a platform and obtaining approvals. "My first job is always to get the parents and teachers to believe in what I'm doing. Then I can get underway. We work with groups of about ten. These young people are great assets in alcohol education. They are exciting to work with and stimulate an interest among fellow students that is unsurpassed by other modes of teaching."

Peer Education effectively helps young people, individually and in groups, to pinpoint their problems, acquire the knowledge that is essential to solve the problems, and then take necessary action. The unique ingredient is the interchange of knowledge between peers that leads to plans of action that have reasonable objectives. Or, as the prospectus for the program describes the approach, it is a matter of "student helping student." "Peer educators," as the young group leaders are called, are trained in techniques of getting through to youth.

Some positive guidelines for establishing rapport are:

- Facilitate trust, openness, comfort, empathy.
- Accept people as they are.
- Listen—physically, mentally, emotionally.
- Clarify alternatives for decision making.
- Give support and encouragement to positive action.
- Respect confidentiality.
- Realize that not all people can be helped.
- Realize that not all problems can be solved.
- Work with young people who have normal, if sometimes acute, growing-up problems.
- Refer the really troubled individuals to a professional, qualified counselor.

Negative actions that peer educators and parents must avoid are:

- Preaching or telling young people what to do.
- Judging people and trying to change them.
- Offering solutions and giving advice.
- Acting as a "rescuer" and doing for a person what he or she should be doing independently.
- Gossiping or putting people down.
- Attempting to work with those who are seriously disturbed and in need of professional help.
- Trying to provide services and counsel beyond what they are qualified to provide.

How does the program work?

"When we get young people together in these sessions where students are helping students," says Terry Royer, "they really open up and are very expressive when the situation is right. Yet some of the kids in the program were originally so backward and reluctant that they would hardly even give their first names, let alone enter into any kind of discussion.

"I know it's asking a lot to expect parents to imagine themselves as participants in this kind of rap session," he says. "But if they could just try to simulate something of the outlooks and approaches, they would accomplish wonders. At the very least, if parents are really hung up, totally jammed when it comes to getting through to a kid in trouble, then they should locate a program in which young people are able to establish this kind of dialogue."

The Boys' Clubs of America have organized a program, Teens Explore Alcohol Moderation (Project TEAM), designed "to encourage young people to make responsible decisions about drinking." They recognize one of the basic challenges: there are manifold influences that lead young people into drinking, but only a handful that are effective in discouraging youthful experimentation. The TEAM program endeavors to bridge the generation gap between participants, ages thirteen to eighteen, and parents. They bring in well-known public figures, such as movie star Dana Andrews, who have publicly acknowledged that they are recovered alcoholics.

"Peer persuasion, rap sessions, and rehabilitation that involve alcoholics who have controlled their drinking are the best ways to fight this problem," said Andrews at one meeting. "A teenager can go from hard drugs to alcohol in six months and become an alcoholic. With an alcoholic there really is no cure. As the saying goes, one drink is too much and one thousand are not enough."

13 | *What do alcohol education programs mean to young people?*

Many adults I have talked with have expressed astonishment on being told about the nature and extent of some of the programs on alcoholism that are available to teenagers, and even to preteenagers, across the country. Some programs have been established specifically to help young people who are already having alcohol-related problems. Other programs are educational and preventive in nature, attended largely by young people who are unfamiliar with alcohol but are certain to be exposed to it in the near future. The formats range from one- or two-hour rap sessions to well-structured conferences that may last for several days.

For instance, the Third Annual Illinois Teenage Institute on Substance Abuse, at a 4-H camp in Monticello, Illinois, lasted five days. According to Gerrit L. DenHartog, executive director of the Illinois Alcoholism and Drug Dependence Association, institute conferences have been highly successful. Using the theme "Life Is Now," the institute underscored the statement "It's your life and your decision" with the idea that each participant has the capacity to base decisions on accurate information and a better understanding of the self and personal motivations.

Successful alcohol education programs seem to favor this concept: teenagers must be presented with sufficient, and pertinent, facts to make their own decisions—not lectured to or told what to do and what attitudes to take.

Carrying this concept one step further, the institutes encourage young people to take follow-up action by developing appropriate activities and initiating helping relationships in their home communities. Such activities mean helping others to follow similar courses of action and getting involved with those who need help. This represents a practical application of the theory that you will strengthen your own belief in something if you have enough conviction to pass it along to others. Among the significant comments of the eighty or so boys and girls, mostly high school juniors or sophomores, were these:

The institute to me was a place where you could speak your feelings without anyone thinking you were weird. The best part was that the speakers did not tell us that certain substances were bad and we should stay away from them. Instead, they gave us the facts and let us make our own decisions.

We talked in detail and in depth. But we did more than that. We got to know and love those around us. When you heard sad stories about alcoholic parents and drug-addicted brothers and sisters, you could really feel for that person.

The sessions gave me the incentive to go back and help people in my community, especially since I now have the background and knowledge necessary to help others.

It was a chance for us young people to talk and discuss whatever was on our minds, openly and without guilt.

I learned much about people—as much in five days as I had in a lifetime.

I found myself and I met the most beautiful people. They *cared*. The institute was the greatest experience of my entire life. I still think of it every day.

Parents are not likely to receive such encomiums from sons and daughters, no matter how skillfully they communicate or develop a rapport on the home front. As one mother said, "If my sixteen-year-old comments that something I've done is 'okay,' I translate that to mean 'super' in terms of the idiom he'd use with his peers." But it is encouraging to know that kids can get what they refer to as a "natural high" through serious discussions of problems and situations that generate problems.

Significant, too, may be the opinion among these young people that the small-group format is excellent and that rap sessions should be short, as well as to the point. Thus, if you are trying to encourage a teenager with a drinking problem to seek help through discussion groups, when you have made little headway with other approaches, steer him in the direction of programs that are brief and well defined.

It is perhaps for this reason that more and more teenagers are showing up in A.A. (Alcoholics Anonymous) meetings these days. Members speak out explicitly about drinking problems, do not wander into other topics, and show little embarrassment in speaking openly about experiences that can be pretty hairy. Young people seem to react well to this directness, accepting a kinship with people who can "tell it like it is." Brevity is often refreshing because they are accustomed to detractors, whether at home, in school, or in the neighborhood who seem to be on their backs, ad infinitum. They are able to surface in the A.A. milieu, rather than have the feeling that they have been dragged to bottomless depths.

What is it like to be at an A.A. meeting?

It is 8:30 on a Tuesday evening. Some thirty people, ranging in age from seventeen to seventy, are seated around or parallel to several tables that have been pushed together to form a large one. The location is a basement room of a church, an area normally used for Sunday school classes. Two or three years ago, the youngest regular attendee was a secretary in her late twenties. Tonight, there are four teenagers, and three or four young adults who seem to be under twenty-five. But age makes no difference here. Neither does sex, race, religion, education, income, social standing, or any of the usual categories by which people are classified.

Most of the people in the room are sipping coffee or tea. Some are smoking. They are chatting, reading booklets, or perhaps just sitting in thought. At the head of the table a woman in her early thirties shuffles some scribbled notes in front of her, glances at a typed sheet, then raps sharply with a pencil on her coffee cup. "I guess we are ready to begin," she says. The conversationalists phase out their chatter, settle back in their seats, and look in her direction.

This is a regular meeting of Alcoholics Anonymous.

The leader for the evening reads the brief creed, which states that A.A. is "a fellowship of men and women who share their experience, strength, and hope with each other that they may solve their common problem and help others to recover from alcoholism. . . .

"The only requirement for membership is a desire to stop drinking. There are no dues or fees for A.A. membership; we are self-supporting through our own contributions."

The creed also emphasizes that A.A. has no affiliations with any sect, denomination, political groups, or other organizations or institutions; neither endorses nor opposes any causes; and does not engage in controversies—not even issues related to alcohol and alcoholism. "Our primary purpose," it concludes, "is to stay sober and help other alcoholics to achieve sobriety."

A typical meeting lasts an hour and a half or two hours. Generally, the leader introduces a speaker, who may be a regular member of the group or from a nearby group. Almost without exception, he or she is an A.A. member who, after an introduction by first name, admits, "I am an alcoholic." The speaker may talk for fifteen or twenty minutes, part of the time recounting past experiences and behavior that resulted directly from hitting the bottle. Then the discussion will shift to a topic for the evening, such as "anonymity," and each member in the room will be given an opportunity to comment, ask questions, or simply remain silent.

No one is ever pressured in any way to speak up. The comment "I'll pass," or "I'm just listening now," is respected. New members may be shy or deeply confused from recent drinking. Older members may really prefer to listen at that moment, or have other reasons for not entering the discussion. Young people who are new to A.A. seem more inclined to open up, ask questions, or describe their experiences than are older people. Possibly this willingness—even urge—to enter into a dialogue stems from recent participation in rap sessions at school or college or in meetings held by various types of youth organizations concerned about attitudes and behavior.

The situation is quite astonishing when you think about it. You plunk a young person of eighteen or nineteen or twenty down in a group of complete strangers—who may be parents, business people, lawyers, doctors, teachers, or members of the clergy—and you expect that person to open up and reveal hair-raising inner secrets that no one else on earth may yet know. Yet it works!

Are there criticisms of A.A.?

Some people have accused A.A. of being "secretive." But there is a marked difference betweeen subterfuge of any kind and the *anonymity* that is practiced by members. The latter is a key factor in making it possible for many problem drinkers to abandon their secretive practices and bring their problems out into the open. This approach apparently has more and more appeal for young people.

The "Early Starters" group, which began as a teenage chapter of A.A. in the Baltimore area several years ago, is aptly named. The participants, ages fifteen to twenty-five, had been drinking when they were still in elementary school. Jan had her first drink at the age of eleven when she discovered her older brother drinking in his bedroom and threatened to snitch on him if he didn't let her sample his beer. By the time she had reached high school, she was "spending a lot of time in the school parking lot with a keg of beer."

Rick was even more precocious. He sampled his first drink at the age of eight and was a full-fledged alcoholic by his fourteenth birthday. His parents put him in the hands of a psychiatrist, not realizing until too late that the doctor himself had a drinking problem and was hardly the one to try to convince a teenager to put the cork back on the bottle. Rick enlisted in the army as the more attractive alternative to flunking courses in school, but lasted only three months, most of that time in a military mental ward.

Jay described his drinking career before joining the Early Starters as a downhill slide from active athlete to student drunkard. For a while, in his early teens, he achieved some notoriety as the youthful adventurer who could be counted on to sneak coolers of beer into the school yard, right under the noses of the faculty. Inevitably, he was caught and expelled.

Patty started "messing around with booze" in the ninth grade and by the time she had reached senior high was also popping pills. She ultimately managed to graduate, but mainly because she was taken abroad when her father was transferred and stayed straight long enough to get a diploma from an American school in Europe.

These are but a few of the thousands of cases of young people who have been able to put themselves back on the road to recovery through A.A. There are no neat formulas for success, no guarantees that the program will work in every case, but it has been indisputably demonstrated that the A.A. approach does get through to many young people with drinking problems, and that the concept of anonymity is a strong factor in getting them started.

How can a peer group help?

If you are unsure of your relationship with a child who evidences drinking problems, if you realize that you have *not* brought up your children to make responsible decisions, or if for any other reason you sense that now you have reached a point of crisis and are not mentally, emotionally, or educationally equipped to handle the situation, you have a strong—possibly unsuspected—ally: the child's own friends, classmates, and other young associates.

Wait a minute! you exclaim. That is the very reason the kid is in trouble. He is hanging out with some buddies who are into booze and leading him on, beyond our control.

A different group of peers may be able to turn the situation around. "The peer group represents a powerful force in shaping and influencing the behavior of others," says John Zachariah. He agrees with almost every professional who works in this field that "the most effective method of limiting alcohol abuse is primary prevention through systematic prevention education." Such education, as in the case of most learning processes, is going to be more productive if it is started in early childhood, during the earliest stages of an individual's psychological development. "This means education beginning in the family . . . through elementary school to adulthood. This is the holistic approach [the belief that an entity is more than simply the sum of tis parts] to developing a responsible community, which in turn will have a positive impact on the development of responsible drinking behavior in its members."

What are some of the ingredients in an educational program?

Alcohol education programs can be simple or complex. Madonna Clifford Fullerton, project director of a program for sixth-, seventh-, and eighth-graders that was tried on an experimental basis at the Maine Health Education Resource Center, University of Maine, said: "As a resident of a rural area in Maine, I am particularly sensitive to the situations of rural people who have problems with alcohol. I am also aware of the deficiency in literature about alcohol abuse as far as those rural problems are concerned." The objective of the program was "to teach our young people about alcohol and to provide them with the skills necessary to make responsible decisions about alcohol use."

An important ingredient in the program's success was the materials used to spark the children's interest in a way that got them involved. Among the more imaginative devices used were slides dramatizing teenagers in trouble because of drinking, as well as role playing and the preparation of "Dear Abby" letters.

The slide shows are based on real-life experiences, to which the young viewers can relate either directly or indirectly (although some parents might consider the situations portrayed as being exaggerated or certainly not based on events occurring in *their* communities). The following example is typical:

("Brenda" is telling her sister, who has been experimenting with a six-pack of beer, why their father had grounded her for three months when she was in the eighth grade.) "He caught me and another kid out in the barn drinking beer. I sure was mad. He drinks beer when he wants to. Mom has wine or a cocktail when she wants to, so why shouldn't I? If it didn't hurt them, I figured it couldn't hurt me. Besides, I thought it was fun getting high. Man, we used to have some crazy parties when someone would get some vodka and spike the punch. Half the kids didn't know we were doing it. It was really fun to watch them get high and not really know what was happening to them. We were just having a good time, or so we figured . . ."

(Not wanting to hear what "Brenda" has to say, the sister, "Anne," tries to get her friend, "Diane," who had seemed a bit cool lately, to come over and drink beer with her. Getting a negative response, she tries to put some pressure on "Diane" by calling her "chicken.")

"Diane" replies: "I said I'm not interested and that's that. If you think that makes me a chicken, then just go find yourself another friend, if you can, and leave me alone. And . . . you say you're as healthy as ever (referring to a comment by Anne that drinking hasn't hurt her) . . . have you taken a good look at yourself lately? If you're so healthy, why did the gym teacher take you off the first team? And why have you been having so many detentions? And why are you flunking science, which was your best subject last quarter? And why do you always look so spaced out?"

(In the end, after various scenes make it clear that "Anne" really felt she had messed up her life to the point of no return, she is convinced that she really has not proved anything by continuing to drink beer, which she started just for kicks.)

"Anne" admits: "It was just an excuse, I guess. I was confused about a lot of things. I didn't understand me any more. I didn't feel like a kid . . . but I found out that I'm not an adult either. I guess the alcohol was an escape from having to try to figure out what was happening to me. The big problem was that as soon as I'd sober up, I'd be depressed because nothing was any clearer than before."

After the film, pupils were asked questions relating to the situations and the people depicted. Samples:

Do you think Anne's reaction in Scene 2 was typical of teenagers in the same situation? Explain.

Brenda said, "Kids are apt to do dumb things when they're drinking." Is this true only of kids? What causes people to do dumb things when they're drinking? Is there any way to avoid having this happen?

How would you evaluate Diane's attitude toward Anne? Do you think she is "chicken" as Anne says?

Why is it important for Anne to realize that one mistake doesn't mean she's a failure as a person?

In answering questions of this kind, children have to apply value judgments that help them develop standards for themselves in relation to alcohol use.

How is role playing used as a technique?

You are hitch-hiking to school when a nice-looking lady in a station wagon offers you a ride. You recognize her as a mother you have seen in the town. After getting into the car, though, you smell whiskey on her breath. It is pretty strong. In the back of the wagon are two small children.

What should you do? Why?

This is one of the questions used in the Maine program, which has been getting productive results. Here are examples of others:

You have tried your parents' liquor while they are out. They come home and find you acting "funny." What happens?

After school, you go home with a friend and find the mother drunk. What, if anything, do you say to your friend? What does the friend do? What does the mother say?

Your class is going on a field trip, for which each student must pay $1.60. You ask your parents, but there is no money in the house because your father has spent it all on drinking. What do you say? What do your parents say?

These are not easy questions to answer. Indeed, there is no specific "correct" answer and no intent to grade pupils. Role playing is not intended as a game, an escape from one's own pattern of life. Rather, it is an admitted device to stimulate participants to think about alcoholic behavior and decision making.

Another effective technique, and a further extension of role playing, is known as the "Dear Abby" approach. Participants are asked to write imaginary letters to the columnist and to come up with what they feel are acceptable answers. Some samples:

Dear Abby:
My father is an alcoholic. It started as a few drinks a night but now he drinks continuously. I love him a lot and I know somebody should help him because he needs help desperately. What should I do?   Need Help

Dear Need Help:

I'm sure there is a place for you to call and get information on what to do. Ask your mother if she can help you. Sit down and explain to her that you want to help him, and if you can ever get your father when he's sober, tell him you care and you love him and you wish he would stop.
Abby

Dear Abby:

I started out drinking just for fun, but later the pressure was so big I started drinking all the time. They showed it on TV, so why can't I? I have problems too.
Hooked on Booze

Dear H.O.B.:

Drinking will hide your problems for now. But sooner or later you're going to have to face them. Find someone you can tell your problems to, so they can help. Try to cut down on the amount you drink until eventually you stop.
Abby

Dear Abby:

My father is an ex-alcoholic. He hasn't touched a drink in five years. Do you think it would hurt him if I drank when I got older? What should I do?
Confused

Dear Confused:

If you do drink, which you shouldn't, don't bring it to the home and don't go home drunk. To answer your question, yes, it will hurt him.
Abby

Is there any follow-up to this program?

"There are no counseling activities within the scope of this program," Ms. Fullerton said. "If a teacher becomes aware of a student who has a drinking problem, then that student is either referred to an appropriate counseling agency or is made aware of possible sources of assistance."

14

Is there a national commitment to alcohol education?

If a young person close to you is taking—or about to take—a course in alcohol education, you will want to know: Is the course any good? Can it really help an adolescent who is in trouble or potentially in trouble because of drinking? Isn't there a danger that the topics discussed might confuse a young person who has never tried booze, or might even suggest some dangerous ideas?

Alcohol education is a relatively new subject. Years ago, as one handbook points out, during the days of Prohibition, the subject was sometimes covered in biology or a health class. The teacher would hold up a bottle showing a worm preserved in alcohol, suggesting that this was what might happen to your internal organs if you drank. The scare tactic had only a fleeting effect because most pupils were intelligent enough to know that the worm was preserved in a potion considerably stronger than what would get into their stomachs if they drank. This educational approach to drinking, especially the use of statistics calculated to alarm rather than to inform, continued pretty much until the 1960s. So it is natural for adults to question the nature and effectiveness of any course labeled "alcohol education."

One of the best recognized authorities in this field is Dr. Gail Milgram, of the Center of Alcohol Studies at Rutgers University. She points out that alcohol education in the United States lacks status; it is inconsistent in content in the same grade level (even in the same geographic area), and is often totally neglected. The reasons for the deficiencies are many.

"There is no national commitment to a program of alcohol education," says Dr. Milgram. "Though most states have program guides or curriculum guides, in most areas their distribution is not a priority, and the majority of regions have no county or community programs to aid such an effort. . . .

"The Temperance Movement, Prohibition, and subsequent Repeal affected society in general and alcohol education specifically in a significant manner. Even though society has changed a great deal from the time of Prohibition, ambivalence still clearly surrounds alcohol use and education."

As she points out, schools are reluctant to face the issue, often letting it be known that abstinence should be stressed, at least until legal drinking age. "However," she says bluntly, "the fact that the majority of our young people are using alcohol prior to legal age is producing a clear quandary for educators."

Not infrequently, the approach to the subject places so much emphasis on the problems and the *ism* in *alcoholism* that young people are quickly turned off. It is only natural for them to fear that if they show interest, they will be labeled alcoholics.

What are the objectives of alcohol education programs?

"The primary objective of alcohol education is to help students to live realistically and responsibly in a society characterized by a wide diversity of attiudes and behavior patterns related to alcoholic beverages."

This statement appears in a resource book for teachers entitled *Learning About Alcohol,* published by the National Education Association, which points out that not all courses go far enough beyond presenting the facts and clearing the air. "Unfortunately," says the guide, "many educational programs are still designed around subjects and grades. A student may score 100 on a test about alcohol; he may immediately celebrate, if he so chooses, by going out and having a beer or two or getting drunk."

Are there any successful alcohol education programs?

Rosemary Carmichael teaches public school and nonpublic school students in the Bronx, the northern borough of New York City. The fact that she is dealing largely with boys and girls in their preteens would seem routine, were it not for the subject: *alcoholism.*

During the past five years, she told me, she has had three times as many referrals to her programs for alcohol-related problems as for those that are drug-related. She has also seen a steady increase in alcohol use and misuse by young people in her area and a change in the boy/girl percentages so that there are now almost as many female as male teenagers experimenting with alcohol. But Carmichael is not concerned only with young people who are heavily on the bottle. Much of her time and work are focused on education and preventive programs designed to reduce alcohol-related problems and reach budding alcoholics before they really get into trouble.

"Young people can be reached at the age level where maturity is taking place and important values are being set," she explains. "One way of reaching the young most effectively is in the elementary school classroom, by providing nonjudgmental, objective information about alcoholic beverages, their potency, and their use."

To accomplish this, she schedules small group discussions, creates a warm, nonthreatening atmosphere in which discussions can be open and frank, and assumes a supportive role in order to help young people get in touch with their feelings and learn more about themselves, as well as about alcohol. Once these groups or "teams" are established and members acquire confidence in themselves, they are introduced to adults from outside the school who are professionals in various fields—police officers, educators, members of Alcoholics Anonymous, doctors and health officials, and others who can speak with authority.

Why do we need an alcohol education program?

"Alcohol education programs form an integral part of the basic education of our youngsters," Carmichael asserts. "The school needs to take a strong stand in this matter for a number of reasons—to show that we care about and support the home and community, to develop a program in which youngsters can perceive the nature of alcohol and alcohol-related problems, to enable young individuals to understand and clarify their values, and to ask them what they think should be done to improve the situation."

Many parents in so-called "conservative" communities may be surprised—even shocked—to learn about the extent of the educational involvement of children who, traditionally and historically, have been overlooked as too young to be concerned about such problems as heavy drinking and alcoholism. Could you pass one of the regular tests given to a typical *sixth-grade* class, whose pupils were asked to reply "True" or "False"* to twenty questions, including the following?

- Alcohol is a drug.
- Because it is a stimulant, alcohol tends to pep a person up.
- Alcohol in quantity will damage organs in the human body.
- You'll get drunker on vodka or gin or rum than on the same amount of whiskey.
- An alcoholic can be helped.
- You can sober up quickly by drinking black coffee and dousing your head with cold water.
- A person can die of alcohol poisoning.
- Everyone's body reacts the same way to the same amount of alcohol.
- Liquor taken straight will affect you faster than liquor mixed with water or soda in a highball.
- Drunkenness and alcoholism are the same thing.

The children are asked to comment voluntarily on their own experiences involving alcohol, as well as on classroom discussions or talks given by guest speakers. How do children in the sixth grade react to an alcohol education session? Some samples:

I used to drink two cans of beer a day. Then I stopped around two months ago. I kept on having the feeling about taking a drink of anything. But I stopped thinking about it. After joining this program I knew what a drink can do to me. Now I am going to stop drinking. I am going to join a group called the Pioneers. My mother and father are in it and now I feel a lot better.

* The correct answers alternate: True, False, True, False, and so on.

I am very interested in this alcohol program because my mother and father's friends drink an awful lot. . . . If my father's friends drink my father will drink so I will have to know more about alcohol because I don't want my parents getting this disease. Once my father got drunk and he had to drive home in his car, but he is okay. Please let me know more.

What I liked about the program was that a lot of questions we had to ask, we got answers to that helped us. Also, I liked the film. It showed me all the things that can happen when you get absolutely drunk. It also showed me that when I grow up and someone says "Here, have a drink," I'll know what will happen if I do.

I've learned how each drug affects you in a different way. I don't think the program needs any changes except for one. You should get more people involved and also stay in each school for more than four weeks—at least stay six weeks.

I liked the program because it was fun. It was educational. The coordinator talked a lot about experiences. I learned a lot that I did not know. We talked about a lot of other things that concerned the use of drugs and alcohol. *We also talked about ourselves.* I did not like the short time we had.

I like the films and I like when you answered our questions. I like when you gave us that period to write questions, then answered some. I like when you tell stories. I didn't like it because periods were short. And you are leaving too soon.

In addition to commenting that the sessions and programs were too short, many of the pupils commented on the ways in which the curriculum has helped them to communicate—with teachers, peers, parents. For example:

I like the program because I can talk about things I couldn't talk about before with my family 'cause I know more.

The program has helped me a lot. After each program I would go home and talk with Mother about what I learned. Me and my mother would discuss it. I think it was worth it.

The alcohol program was very educational. I most of all loved the way the coordinator communicated and gave us examples of things that happen every day. I liked the way the teachers helped us to understand that drugs and alcohol are very serious problems and they are also killers!

Before I took the program I had a hard time talking with my mother and father about alcohol and didn't talk about it. But when you learn about alcohol you can talk about it and that's what I do when I go home.

I got a lot out of the fact sheet and question sheet that I did not know. I showed them to my father one day and he was very interested. He asked me what we learned and I told him about the film, too. The man was hitting the woman all the time because he was drinking. Alcohol problems can be solved, though, and I told my mother what we had learned about them.

This program told me about the dangers of alcohol and what I can do to get help. It can help me help someone else and teach them what the program taught me.

Do children this young need alcohol education programs?

"One of the important things we have ourselves learned," Rosemary Carmichael told me, "is that schools must start their alcohol education programs in elementary school. Equally important, parents must realize that if they wait until their children are teenagers before giving any thought to telling them about alcohol, they may be too late."

Although this viewpoint might have been controversial a decade ago, it is now being accepted and expressed by teachers and counselors all over the country. "Parents have to be far more alert about alcohol, beginning when children are in the fifth and sixth grades," warns Dr. Gail Milgram. "Junior high school is too late."

Magazine and newspaper articles have overreacted, however, to statements like this, implying that youngsters are drinking at earlier and earlier ages. They miss the point. The importance of reaching fifth- and sixth-graders is to provide instruction and information at a time when their young minds are ready to assimilate such knowledge and understand the subject at hand. Teachers no longer consider sex education, for example, as something that should be withheld until a student reaches junior or senior high school.

Gary Fair is of the opinion that "we do teenagers a disservice by suddenly focusing attention on their lack of knowledge about alcoholism—after having neglected to tell them any-thing about it when they were in their preteens."

Parents who are fortunate enough to live in school districts where alcohol education programs reach children of ten or eleven should do all they can to find out about the course of in-struction, support it, and if necessary take steps to see that it is continually reviewed and improved. But what do you do if you have children in this age group and live in a district where no such instruction is available?

Your first step must be to find out *why* an alcohol educa-tion program is nonexistent. Perhaps no one in authority realizes that this kind of curriculum is necessary. Worse yet, there may be active opposition to such a program, just as there has been to sex education in elementary schools in the past. It may not be easy to generate interest in a course for preteenagers, even with help from agencies and organizations in the area whose con-cerns and functions relate to alcohol and other drugs.

If no resources are available, parents can institute their own family discussions on alcohol, preferably with the help of an outside counselor. The average parent is in the Dark Ages in this sensitive subject area and is likely to believe as many myths as facts about drinking.

Are children at the fifth- and sixth-grade level likely to think of subjects related to drinking as being humorous? silly? embarrassing? Not at all. Rosemary Carmichael has found that her young pupils (many of whom are not the best pupils when it comes to more traditional subjects) take a keen interest in the subject of alcohol, quickly lose their image of a drunk as being funny (if they had this opinion to begin with), and ask intelli-gent questions. One of her fifth-grade pupils, age ten, took the initiative and compiled a list of thirty-five questions asked of a member of Alcoholics Anonymous who had come to address the class during one of the regular "visitation" hours that are held each week. Here is a sample:

- Why did you want to drink?
- Did you drink more as you got older?
- Why do you think you wanted to get away from the world?

- When you stopped drinking, did your family love you more?
- If you didn't have a family, do you think you would have stopped drinking?
- Did your children know how much you were drinking and what you were doing?
- If you owned a pet, do you think the animal would notice anything strange about you when you drank?
- Did you ever feel embarrassed or strange in front of your friends because you drank too much?

Another student in Ms. Carmichael's program, age twelve, narrated a creditable—and credible—tape on the subject, "An Escape from Reality." She explored questions about why people drink, why they think they are having fun or going along with the crowd, and why people are sheeplike in their susceptibility to slogans like "Try It—You'll Like It." She also convincingly compared alcoholism to a fever that increases and spreads within the body until the patient has little control over his physical or mental capabilities. Then she concluded:

"Let's have courage to say *no* and *yes—no* to the desire to escape from the world and *yes* to the person you are, the person you want to be, and the person God expects you to be."

Parents are often pleasantly surprised at the degree of interest and soundness of their youngsters' response. Counselors have told me that they have little, if any, difficulty getting kids involved in programs. Several have said, however, that when it comes to parents, quite a few are reluctant to participate—or even to have their children enrolled in alcohol education programs.

All of the successful alcohol education programs establish goals that include the endeavor to help young people understand and clarify their values in regard to alcohol and to have their behavior reflect their values. The objectives are to help young people get in touch with their feelings in order to learn about themselves; to show them how to live realistically and responsibly in a society characterized by a wide diversity of attitudes related to alcoholic beverages; to develop their sense of responsibility for their own well-being and that of others; and to strengthen their capacity to stand by their own convictions, even if it sometimes means ostracism and isolation.

Along with the hard facts and figures, young people can discover much about their outlooks and beliefs. "I knew more about booze than Hiram Walker does," asserted a fifteen-year-old, "because I was shaping my life-style around drinking—and drunks. But until I joined the Alc Ed group I never knew that a guy could drink and be civilized at the same time."

Why are so few educators involved in alcohol programs?

Most programs have been launched by professional counselors in the field of alcoholism, or even by recovered alcoholics who are trying to spare young people some of the miseries they endured. Public school adminstrators and educators have avoided involvement—whether deliberately or otherwise—because they are not trained for this field. On the subject of alcohol the average educator is likely to have a too general overview, if he has one at all.

Because it is a new field, few educators are aware of the different kinds of needs at different age levels when it comes to the matter of alcohol use. Elementary school pupils, for example, wonder why people drink this unfamiliar and foul-tasting substance which (if they have tried it at all) seems more like a medicine than a drink. The junior high student is likely to have questions that indicate a personal curiosity: What are the various beverages? How strong are they? What will each one do to me if I drink it?

The high school student may have similar questions but is likely to be more concerned about the unattractive disease of alcoholism, legal matters, and how dangerous it is to drive after having a couple of beers or cocktails. Any curriculum that ignores such needs and attempts to present alcohol as one subject will have serious deficiencies.

Educators often feel uncomfortable in trying to introduce the subject into the general curriculum. "Many teachers, parents, and school administrators are understandably reluctant to involve the school in teaching youngsters about human behavior in an area as sensitive and personal as alcohol use," explains a guide for elementary school teachers published by the National Council on Alcoholism. "Such concern often stems from the belief that talking about alcohol promotes drinking by inciting youngsters' curiosity; that education dealing with personal behavior is the responsibility and prerogative solely of parents; and that encouraging teachers to discuss alcohol puts many of them in the uncomfortable position of feeling they have to conceal their own drinking behavior."

Many communities apparently are concerned also that teachers and counselors who are assigned to the subject may then feel that they have been given license to impose their own drinking standards and codes on the students in their charge.

No matter how well organized a school program may be, it is limited by the viewpoint of the individual teachers who must try to resolve the confusions and contradictions. Society approves of adult use of alcohol in moderation, but generally frowns on use by teenagers. As a result, teachers are likely to take the stance that adult use is sanctioned but use by young people is hazardous, if not illegal. This places the instructor in the unenviable position of endorsing a double standard, thus weakening his ability to carry on an effective dialogue.

Should alcohol education be taught with drug education?

Some educators argue that the problem of alcohol abuse is the number one concern today, as compared with several years ago when the use of other drugs rated top consideration. Therefore, they rationalize, by lumping the two subjects together the seriousness of alcohol abuse is de-emphasized. *The Journal of School Health* reported that "25 percent of all seventh-graders report getting drunk one or more times a year" and that "twenty-five percent of all high school students report they get drunk four or more times a year." By comparison, says the article, "teenage abuse of other drugs is much less widespread." Only 3.6 percent of a national sampling of more than 12,000 junior and senior high school students had used a "hard" drug like heroin or cocaine during a six-month test period.

Another argument in favor of keeping the two subjects separate in the classroom is that most Americans, as has already been noted, view the moderate use of alcohol as an acceptable social practice while few condone the use of other drugs, moderately or otherwise. "Alcohol education has as its goal," says the *Journal*, "not abstinence but responsible decision making about alcohol. Whether students choose to drink as adults (or even as children) in socially acceptable and legally sanctioned circumstances is their decision. A goal of drug education is to discourage students from using other drugs at all for nonmedical purposes."

15

What role do churches play in alcohol education?

In the summer of 1977 an article appeared in *Alcohol Health and Research World* under the title, "The Church and Alcoholism: A Growing Involvement." At about the same time, those attending a meeting of the National Council on Alcoholism in San Diego were being told by a minister that many members of the clergy tend *not* to get involved in the issues of alcoholism because of the inhibiting attitudes they hold.

Which outlook is prevalent?

This is certainly one area where you should be able to expect assistance and at least counsel if you are concerned about young people with drinking problems. A poll taken by the Louis Harris organization in 1974 reported that 87 percent of the people queried felt that the clergy should play a more important role in helping and advising problem drinkers of all ages. The survey, taken on behalf of the National Institute on Alcohol Abuse and Alcoholism, clearly indicated that people *want* their churches to become more involved in alcohol problems.

Yet, says the editorial, "some people see the negative emotional attitude of many Americans toward alcohol consumption as something that has been nurtured by the church. They feel that this attitude is particularly intense in America because of the active role religious groups played in the powerful temperance movement that spearheaded the drive to achieve national prohibition."

Even more destructive may be the abstinence stance of some churches, which interprets alcohol and alcoholism in terms of "moral" issues. As has been discussed earlier, the moralistic and judgmental approach to drinking problems, especially among youth, has been a disruptive and harmful factor rather than a beneficial one.

The Reverend Karl A. Schneider, director of education at the Eagleville, Pennsylvania, Hospital and Rehabilitation Center, says that there are "attitudinal stumbling blocks" which must be overcome before any minister can successfully administer to problem drinkers. Few members of the clergy have received adequate training, if any, in counseling young people with alcohol or drug problems.

In my own experience, I encountered one situation that disturbed me at the time. A number of publications mentioned that I was compiling this book and suggested that readers who might have material of interest get in touch with me. The most productive mention was a short article that appeared in a monthly newsletter, published by the National Institute on Alcohol Abuse and Alcoholism, which is mailed free to anyone concerned with alcohol and alcoholism. It generated several hundred inquiries, many of which led to valuable contacts and the development of pertinent information and quite a few productive discussions and dialogues. But out of all those inquiries, only *five* came from members of the clergy or church-oriented groups.

This was hardly a scientific survey, yet it gave the impression that few churches are actively involved in a practical way with educating young people about drinking and the nature of alcohol and alcoholism. I expressed this belief one evening to a group of five young people, following a regular meeting of Alcoholics Anonymous. All were A.A. members, ranging in age from eighteen to mid-twenties. Here are some of their comments:

LIZ: This happens to be my church. We have A.A. meetings here twice a week and the pastor opens the doors for meetings by, and for, young people. There is also, I think, a regular group which comes here to discuss the drug scene—other than alcohol as a drug. But the church itself does not seem to have much involvement. For example, I have never seen the pastor at an A.A. meeting—an open one, that is, to which he would be welcome.

ELENA: My church has weekly youth forums, for kids in junior high and high school, on a whole bunch of subjects. I went to one just a couple of weeks ago, which was announced as being on teenage drinking. We had a supper and then a speaker, who was from

our local family consultation service. He passed around some literature for us to take home, all on marijuana. Then he talked for about
an hour. Half of it was on alcohol. But he turned the kids off because
he said the same things we have been hearing right along—all the
horror stories about accidents and suicides and divorces that are
caused by drinking. I didn't get anything out of it at all.

KEVIN: But the church *did* get involved. It wasn't really your
church's fault that the speaker turned out to be so one-sided. Isn't
that what counts?

ELENA: That's one of the points I want to make. The church
really wasn't involved. It simply made arrangements—the guy, the
meal, the hall, the audience. There was no sequence, no follow-up.
The next week the youth forum was on, let's say honor codes and
cheating, and the week after that on attitudes about sex.

KEVIN: Our church has a strong program for helping alcoholics
and families that are in trouble because some member is into the
booze. It's called AID and is run by three deacons who are—or at
least I know two of them are—recovering alcoholics. Also, in the
lobby where there are racks holding church pamphlets and tracts,
there are also several publications from A.A., the National Council
on Alcoholism, and other agencies. It's all there. You can get help.
But I guess what we're driving at as we rap about all this is that
there is really no *youth* program, no educational program.

COOKIE: That seems to be it in my experience. A lot of sym-
pathy from the church and people, and assistance when the going
gets really tough. But not much you could call preventive. It's like a
hospital that has an emergency room but forgot to set up any facilities for giving regular physical exams and advising people on how
to live properly and avoid illnesses.

LIZ: You know, I think our problem here is one—well, it's not
typical. We're in an "affluent" county, where people are supposed to
know these things and get all kinds of help and education on their
own. I was a volunteer in an inner-city project two years ago. Real
ghetto stuff, in the slums. We worked with a black minister in a
church where the congregation was largely blacks and Hispanics.
That man was something else again. He laid it on the line about
drinking. Every man, woman, and child in the congregation was educated about booze. Fire and brimstone stuff. But, you know, it
wasn't "preachy." It was from the heart. I'd say he was involved,
that church was involved. And there must be many other churches
in urban areas like this where the ministers definitely try to do something about alcohol and drinking problems.

MARCIA: My church has a new program which is too new to

provide much of an example. The minister and assistant minister and some of the lay people who work in the church are going to an NCA program on alcoholism. And they have a workshop scheduled for early summer at a camp, where they will meet with other church people—I guess nonchurch groups, too. I know about this because my father is one of the people taking the course. He got into it because of my drinking. So he's personally involved. But, like I said, this is something new—too new to have helped me when I really started to get into the booze two or three years ago.

COOKIE: If you want an overall opinion, from kids I've talked with and things I've seen or had experience with, I think that the church is very timid about anything to do with booze. Probably because ministers really do not know much about the subject. I don't care what church—Catholic, Protestant, Jewish—and of course some churches just shut their ears and ban any kind of drinking and practically don't recognize that there is a disease called alcoholism.

What are some characteristic church programs?

I talked with Father Gregory, a young Boston priest in his late twenties who is in A.A. and had been drinking for five years in an uncontrollable manner before he was able to get sober. He agreed that most clergymen lack the proper education to provide any meaningful counsel to young members of the parish. However, he felt that the Roman Catholic Church was very heavily committed to programs—both preventive and restorative —through its involvement with lay organizations in the field of alcoholism.

Brother Mike Phillips, pointing to the parochial school system in Pittsburgh, emphasized that the Catholic Church itself is involved in many ways although laymen do not give the church credit—or overlook the church's role. An example is his own driver education course, with its focus on the SOBER theme throughout the southwestern Pennsylvania region (see Chapter 7).

It is a healthy sign that clergymen themselves are starting to speak up. "The time has come for churches to move beyond the range of the 'sick alcoholic,'" said the Reverend David A. Works, an Episcopal priest who is president of the North Conway Institute in Boston. Among the areas that churches should concern themselves with, he asserts, are the education of young people regarding the use and abuse of alcohol, the need for more objective information about alcoholic beverages and their effects, and the need to change the attitudes of people about alcoholism.

"Well, there's always the Salvation Army," quipped a woman in her mid-fifties. "I know a couple of soul-savers who could straighten out these kids who tipple!"

Don't laugh. If you are frustrated no matter where you turn for help for a young person, if your own church has an insipid or negative outlook, if the local school program is limited or non-existent—try the Salvation Army. "No other agency or institution, religious or secular, can equal the sheer volume of services that the Salvation Army has rendered to alcoholism throughout the world," said a report by Paul C. Conley and Andrew A. Sorenson on church involvement in this field.

Whether you are a Methodist or not, you can seek help through the United Methodist Church, which maintains an active department of drug and alcohol concerns. It is especially involved with youth through such activities as a curriculum guide on alcohol education for use in teaching students from ninth to twelfth grade and the publication of guides, such as *Alcohol and You*, directed at young readers.*

These new church programs face an enormous challenge just in getting themselves established and attracting young people. They first have to overcome generations of inertia, indifference, and—most deadly—an ingrown genius for turning off youth. Gary Fair related the comments of an associate working with kids who were involved in drugs. When asked if these youngsters had any belief in God, he stated that, of the thousand or so addicts he had worked with, almost all of them believed in God. On the other hand, only a third of them had any use for the church itself. Why should this be so? Three reasons were given:

1. "The kids find church boring and feel the people aren't aware of the real world. . . . The kids feel God is alive and dynamic, but they feel that the church is inactive and dead."

* Pamphlets and other publications available through The Department of Alcohol and Drug Concerns, Division of General Welfare, The United Methodist Church, 100 Maryland Avenue, N.E., Washington, DC 20002.

2. "They feel the church is full of hypocrites," because Christianity teaches forgiveness but that is the last thing the members of the church are likely to give. They will not forget either, and are likely to hold up young people who step out of line as being examples of sinners.

3. "The kids feel that time is of the essence, while the church takes the opposite approach." Churches and parishioners do a great deal of foot dragging, while those who desperately need help continue to suffer.

Fortunately, not all churches have this kind of record today.

According to the National Institute on Alcohol Abuse and Alcoholism (NIAAA), "Young people with addiction problems are the special target of Teen Challenge, a program affiliated with the General Council of the Assemblies of God." The program includes outreach, rehabilitation, education, and help in getting back into a normal society. Young people with problems find their way into the program through drop-in centers, coffee houses, and a hot-line service run by volunteers.

In the words of the study undertaken for the NIAAA, "Local churches across the nation, disturbed by the effect of alcohol abuse on their communities, have initiated a variety of programs to combat the problem." Not all of these are youth-oriented, and not all have yet achieved any real track record. Yet you should look to your church if you have not yet done so and the problem is getting out of hand. "Many parents do not even bother to approach their pastor for help," says the Reverend Benjamin D., a recovering alcoholic who has just been assigned by the Reformed Church to develop an alcohol education program in New England, "because the church has presented such a stuffy and nonhelpful attitude in the past. You might be surprised—and relieved—to know that quite a few things have been going on, sometimes behind closed doors, in parishes all over. Perhaps in yours.

"One of the advantages to you is that alcohol programs, whether to dispense information or meet crises head on, tend to be ecumenical. That is, they cross sectarian boundaries in a way few other activities have ever done. If your church has little to offer, you need have no second thoughts about entering the doors of a church of another denomination. You will be welcome. In fact, there is even some mixing of participants between Christian churches and synagogues."

And Reverend D. adds, "In one way, ironically perhaps, alcoholism is helping to improve interdenominational tolerance and respect in a way that I have never seen in some three decades of ministry."

This is characteristic of most programs concerned with the problems of teenage drinking. People with problems are welcome, no questions asked. Go now—don't wait for an invitation or a membership card!

16 | How are law-enforcement agencies involved with youthful drinking?

"Recent teenage drinking in small towns and large cities throughout the nation is being pinpointed as the basis for most juvenile violence, vandalism, and disrespect for authority," stated Rosemary Carmichael, quoting for me a paper she had delivered at the Rutgers Summer School of Alcohol Studies on the correlation between drinking and law breaking among the young.

"Much criticism is now directed against schools for their indifference to alcohol education, and against local authorities for indifference," she said, "and the courts have been negligent in dealing with youths arrested for crimes that are alcohol-related."

Perhaps you have seen some of the evidence in your own community: increases in arrests for vandalism; the defacement of school buildings, libraries, local monuments, and cemeteries; and empty bottles and crushed beer cans scattered around locations where young people have been gathering. In many areas, the more serious crimes of burglary, break-ins, and violent acts against individuals have increased in direct ratio to the increase in drinking on the part of young people who inhabit those neighborhoods.

"Law enforcement must play a more vital role as well as being included as a discussion topic in an alcohol education program, and it must be of a priority nature," says Rosemary Carmichael, emphasizing that mass-arrest procedures have had minimal results. "Young people must be made to understand that crimes committed while drunk will not be excused because of their condition at the time. Although this approach seemingly has minimal motivating force, the awareness of it might someday be reflected in a reduction of drinking behavior on the part of some."

What is the main focus of law enforcement?

No aspect of the law, as it relates to drinking, receives more attention from professionals of all types than driving. Educators, counselors, doctors, health officials, lawyers, the police, the clergy—all focus on the tragedies and horrors that result. Yet, says Carmichael, "For too long police have taken only minor steps in offering youths their expertise in this vitally needed area. It is common knowledge to most police officers that fatalities caused by drunken-driving youths resulted from alcohol situations that were recognizable before the tragedies occurred. Many officers have spent sleepless nights pondering the question 'What might I have done to prevent that from happening?' "

Many schools have driver education programs that clearly point out to students the effects of alcoholic beverages on a driver's capabilities, reactions, and judgment. Yet policemen and other law-enforcement representatives are usually absent from the classroom, at a time when their presence could count most. Unfortunately, they seldom come into the picture until a young driver has violated traffic laws or become an accident victim because of alcohol abuse. Although the main focus of law enforcement should be on *prevention*, it is on discipline.

Do law-enforcement agencies support youthful programs?

Many programs have started with dialogue, gone on to response, to action—and back to dialogue. Along the way, delinquency has necessarily become a subject of great concern. One program heavily involved in trying to develop correctional, as well as educational, activities is called TADAY (Treatment and Direction for Alcoholic Youth), established in Baltimore in late 1976 for boys and girls, ten to eighteen, whose own alcohol use or that of a family member results in problem behavior. TADAY, explains the project director, Phyllis S. Magnus, "provides an assessment of the extent of alcohol use by the individual and family and offers individualized treatment plans, including individual and group counseling, alcohol education groups, and family counseling."

Many of the young people in the program have had serious enough brushes with the law to be referred to TADAY by the Baltimore City Police Department, Juvenile Court, or other agencies that come under the Law Enforcement Assistance Administration. Once accepted in TADAY, youths are not permitted to enroll in any other treatment program, although the staff often coordinates its work with other groups.

Although TADAY is unique to the Baltimore area and youthful participants must be legal residents of the city, there may be a similar arm of assistance in your area. Such organizations and services are becoming more commonplace as the finger of suspicion points more and more to alcohol abuse as a serious factor in juvenile delinquency and almost every kind of crime in which young people are involved.

The CASPAR program in Somerville, Massachusetts (see Chapter 17), maintains a direct tie-in with all local law-enforcement bodies. In fact, six of the kids in the program recently *conducted* a training session for Somerville police cadets. Picture the role-playing scene, as described by one observer: "Kids are drinking on the corner. The cruiser approaches. The kids played the cops, the cadets played the kids. Sparks flew and nobody wanted to leave. Everybody had faced the session with anxiety at an all-time high, but when it was over the peer leaders reported that it 'went all wrong.' They were shocked at how much they sympathized with the tough role a policeman sometimes has to play. No one would be surprised if some of the cadets, now patrolmen, feel comparably empathetic as they are called upon to disperse kids from street corners."

Are these counseling services sponsored by law-enforcement agencies?

Elva Herzog talked about an innovative counseling service offered in part through the New Jersey Law Enforcement Planning Agency and in part through her township. "The goal of the program," she says, "is to intervene when a youngster has his or her first police involvement, thus reducing the number of repeat offenders."

In most jurisdictions in the United States, juveniles who are arrested for offenses that are alcohol-related are required to attend special classes. The objective is usually to head off later offenses by educating youths about alcohol and attempting to take steps to get them off the booze and hence out of trouble. Sometimes it works; often it does not.

A new approach involves one or both parents. A rural county in Tennessee is doing this effectively. An eight-session "juvenile school" is operated by the Jackson Area Council on Alcoholism and Drug Dependency (JACOADD) as part of a program that includes counseling and remedial education for youngsters who have gotten themselves into trouble through booze. During the classes, youths and parents jointly explore their attitudes toward alcohol after receiving information on the subject. The curriculum also counsels adults and youths alike on ways to improve communications.

Thus far, says David Delmastro, education coordinator for JACOADD, there has been a low rate of repeat offenders among the youths (mainly from fourteen to eighteen) who have attended the school. "We are attempting to provide young people with achievement opportunities," says Delmastro, "to move them toward socially approved goals, and to develop constructive human relationships."

The required attendance by parents is viewed as a vital ingredient in the program's success, since it involves them directly in their children's problems, enhances communications between youths and adults, and improves interfamily relationships.

What if a parent fails to attend a session, or refuses on the grounds that the problem was brought on by the child himself and he is the one who must face the music? Tough luck! The parent can be cited for contempt of court.

"Your child can fool around with alcohol," said one parent, "and you can take positive steps to find a solution. But you cannot fool around with the courts—or you're in deep trouble."

Are counselors knowledgable about the legal implications?

The Reverend Michael J. Miyo serves as an alcoholism counselor in Trenton, New Jersey, for Aid to Low-Income Alcohol Abusers (ALIAA), which has helped a great many teen-agers in trouble with the law. "I see many young people referred to me by the Division of Motor Vehicles, which has an alcohol countermeasures program," he told me, "and also from PTI—Pre-Trial Intervention. Typical comments I hear are 'If only I had known!' or 'If only I had been made aware!' "

A number of factors contribute to both alcohol abuse and steps necessary to help kids once they are in serious trouble. "I have found," says Father Miyo, "that young people do not communicate their problems because they fear the angry re-action that might ensue. Parents, for their part, are often too busy to heed warning signals or do not become concerned until it is too late to avoid serious trouble. Also, if a parent himself has a drinking problem, he will minimize the child's problems—perhaps not even wanting to hear about them. Or he may be at the opposite end of the pole—closing his eyes because he looks upon alcoholism as a stigma or social disgrace.

"The young people I work with tend to have the best rapport with their peers and with some teachers and the poorest rapport with their parents. All of my own patients claim, for example, that one of the problems of relating to parents is the 'double standard'. . . . The kinds of programs that are the most effective and should be brought to the attention of parents are Alateen (nationwide) and Teen Challenge (local) in Rochester, New York."

Reverend Miyo says that to be successful—both to keep young people out of trouble and to assist them after they do get into trouble—a program needs four major ingredients:

1. Proper education about alcoholic beverages and their potency and drinking behavior.

2. Proper education about problem drinking and alco-holism as a disease.

3. Active participation by parents in school and community programs to a degree that will enable them to keep in touch with their children and other young people and make adequate re-ferrals when they themselves find that they cannot cope with a difficult situation.

4. Continuing parental concern, in a caring way, about the

habits of their children and the character and behavior of young people with whom they associate.

"These factors," he says, "will help to keep young people from brushes with the law, or other kinds of alcohol-related troubles."

17 How much can a well-developed community program accomplish?

"Ask many adults in Somerville, Massachusetts, what they think of kids," says Lena DiCicco, "and the odds are they'll complain at some point about the street-corner drinking, the litter of bottles and cans, and the property destruction or harassment they identify with drunk teenagers."

She knows full well what she is talking about. She is director of CASPAR, the Cambridge and Somerville Program for Alcoholism Rehabilitation, which started in July, 1974, in this densely populated city of 89,000 near Boston.

Somerville is probably not much different from many other American cities and towns in the way in which it is faced with a pattern of teenage drinking. The real difference lies in the community's attempts to minimize the incidence of youthful alcoholism. The CASPAR alcohol education program began with a single workshop made up of teachers, guidance counselors, and administrators, under the leadership of Lena DiCicco and Dixie Mills of the Cambridge-Somerville Mental Health and Retardation Center.

The cold front of resistance that usually characterizes initial attempts to discuss alcohol use and abuse was not present in Somerville. Happily, community support was solidly mobilized; the school administration readily accepted and supported the program; and selected high school students were trained to become peer leaders, or alcohol educators, capable of reaching their classmates in a number of settings and circumstances.

A major concern to the founders of the CASPAR program was—as it should be to any community program—the quality of the education. "Ineffective alcohol education is worse than none

155

at all," says the CASPAR report. "By ineffective, we mean it leads the student to come away with a view of alcohol which is even more exaggerated than he or she had before the course, a view which sees alcohol as a mysterious and powerful substance which adults use all the time but tell young people to abhor." Approaches that preach abstinence or stress the consequences of alcohol abuse ignore the value of presenting positive models of behavior.

Individual teacher reactions to participation in the program and the learning experience indicate how their own attitudes were changed by it:

I am now more aware of when, where, and how I drink.

Before, I felt guilty about taking a drink to relax or unwind. Now I know it's a legitimate use of alcohol. I no longer feel pressured to drink or pressure others to drink.

We are more able to cope with the subject when we learn that few people drink without some kind of feelings that they must defend, conceal, minimize, exaggerate, deny, or regulate their drinking on one occasion or another.

Before taking the CASPAR course, I was completely opposed to the lowering of the legal drinking age. I still do not like it, but I am convinced that if teenagers were given proper alcohol education courses, they would become more responsible drinkers.

Most adults favor abstinence as the message to get across to teens. Now I can see why this approach is hypocritical, insulting, and false when measured against the normal teen experience. No sensible student will buy this kind of bias.

Before completing the workshop, I felt that it was important to teach about the bad aspects of alcohol, use all the scare tactics. Now I realize how stupid that viewpoint is.

When I turned my own profile down low, I was better able to stimulate productive student discussions.

This method of teaching has given me new dimensions for interacting with students—and all people—in everyday life.

I learned that we must not overlook the problems of those

students who are deeply affected by alcoholism in their families, but we must realize that most of the kids we are concerned with simply need an education, not personal counsel.

Stressing alcoholism in a general course in alcohol education is like focusing on accidents in driver ed or venereal disease in a sex course.

The teachers in the CASPAR curriculum are, of course, vital ingredients in the achievements that have been recorded since the start of the experiment in the summer of 1974. What should interest you most, however, and what will certainly surprise you, is that much of the success is attributed to the "peer leader" system, whereby teenagers themselves project the image of the program, encourage participation by students, and get involved in the whole information process. The peer leaders perform another valuable function that was not originally anticipated: they occasionally attend adult meetings (such as those of CASPAR's board of directors), where they help immeasurably to make the point that teenagers can be highly responsible and thoroughly motivated in this very sensitive field.

Most peer leaders are "average kids, several of whom have had their share of trouble, their nights of riot and ruin, their E's and F's in school." They know many things about the learning process that adults do not know, so much so that even the teachers are attentive to their suggestions and efforts.

"The responsibilities we give to our peer leaders," says Lena DiCicco, "are to learn, and continue to learn, about alcohol, to practice group techniques that will stimulate discussion and participation, to lead a variety of alcohol education studies and activities, and to serve as an informal network for information and resources."

They are, in effect, educators, yet in a far better position than most professional teachers to get their peers to talk honestly and openly about drinking.

Moreover, they receive recognition in a tangible form—not simply praise, but pay, on an hourly basis, which has the end result of solidifying their relationships with professional adults and earning the respect of classmates.

The special functions of peer leaders are:

• They must interpret the special needs of young people for the benefit of teachers two or three times their age.
• They act as guinea pigs in testing new materials or methods of orientation.
• They are expected to be creative enough to develop effective texts for their peers and come up with a variety of teaching aids that may include puppets, comics, videotapes, role playing, and workshops.
• They have to investigate highly personal and sensitive relationships, yet still respect confidences and shield anonymity.
• They have to resolve questions that are contradictory, like convincing the child of an alcoholic that drinking can be positive, if not beneficial, in many instances.
• They are constantly battling adult disapproval over drinking among the young, while at the same time trying to alleviate the hang-ups and conflicts of their peers.

If you are trying to cope with a teenage drinker or are thinking of becoming involved in a community-action program on teenage drinking, you might keep some of these factors in mind as you ponder the idea of drafting guidelines. You can write CASPAR for its evaluations and progress reports.*

What resources are available in your community?

Alcohol programs in colleges have been proliferating during the last decade. Generally, though, they serve only the student body. One exception is the program inaugurated by the Dallas County Community College District (DCCCD), a system of seven college campuses located within the Dallas, Texas, metropolitan area and serving some 35,000 credit students and a like number of community service students. The philosophy of the college is to "meet community needs with community expertise." Consistent with this philosophy, the DCCCD began in 1977 to expand its internal alcoholism facilities and instruction to provide off-campus assistance for individuals and groups, including young people.

* CASPAR, Inc., 226 Highland Avenue, Somerville, MA 02143.

As part of the activities to make the community aware of drinking problems, an Alcohol Awareness Day was held on each campus, using the theme "Drunk Is Dumb." This was followed a few months later with a "Booze: You Choose" Day, during which some four thousand helium-filled balloons, with slogans such as "Try a Natural High," were given away. Evidence of interest among young people was shown by the fact that almost six thousand students participated in the events of the day.

Well and good, but how does this relate to your problems if you don't happen to live in Dallas County? The development and success of the program indicate that adults concerned about general and specific alcohol-related problems among youth may be overlooking an important resource: local community colleges and other higher-education institutions that have mounted internal alcohol education programs. It is only a short, logical step from campus to community. The citizens who start a dialogue this year to enlist the aid and cooperation of such resources may benefit from the aid available next year.

"Community colleges seem to be both philosophically and practically an ideal setting for community alcohol education programing," reports Vic Shaw, alcohol education specialist at Richland College, Dallas, quoting from a paper he prepared on the Dallas experiment. "The community college's intimate ties with business, politics, industry, and education make it ideally suited to serve the community in the area of alcohol education.

"Residents with alcohol-related problems seem to be more willing to seek help at a 'college' than at a traditional alcoholism clinic or elsewhere. There seems to be less of a social stigma in asking help from a college counseling service than from other counseling services."

As a result of this pioneering step, which is more than likely to spread to other regions, one entire county now has workshops, counseling, rap sessions, and other activities and resources available for people of all ages—but especially the young—who need help because of problems with booze.

Is the situation ever hopeless?

It is almost never too late. A couple of concerned adults can motivate their entire community to develop an alcohol education and assistance program if they have a mind to. This was not true a generation ago, and was barely possible a decade ago. But there are now sufficient organizations and enough well-qualified individuals to make it possible. You will have to listen to the doubters and cynics who moan:

An alcohol education program in our *school system?* Don't start counting the days. The last time an innovative plan was pushed through under protest, it required seven years for the school board to get the rust out of their wheels.

Would the *church* sponsor it? Never. If the minister and his elders had their way, we'd be back in Prohibition days.

So maybe it's the most active program going in some *youth organizations,* but not around here. Ours are nothing more than teen-age clubs interested in softball, bowling, and cook-outs. Try something serious and the members will all quit.

Alcohol and drug organizations? Sure they'd be interested, but only if the community shows sufficient support, and that would be a long time from now.

Faced with community resistance and problems of immediate concern on the home front, parents may logically feel that the best course of action is to seek individual, personal help. There is no doubt that they *can* achieve results, oftentimes through dependable agencies like the Family Consultation Service or local chapters of the National Council on Alcoholism. Moreover, nothing should stop or delay parents from seeking this kind of help. Yet, where young people in particular are concerned, there can be no program so effective during adolescent years as one in which the entire school, perhaps the entire community, is involved. "Teeners make poor loners," said one counselor, "and it is sometimes better to be in a little bit of trouble and in good company than in no trouble in no company."

Should you ever give up
on a teenage drinker?

You may think a son or daughter is hopeless if the young person in question is drinking heavily and has encountered more problems than you ever thought possible—mental, moral, physical, legal, educational, right across the board. Consider, then, the case of "Lana," whose story is on record in the files at the headquarters of Alcoholics Anonymous in New York City.

Lana started drinking at the age of eleven at a wedding, where she seemed to discover an instant friend in the form of champagne. By the time she was thirteen, she was drinking "regularly," on weekends, or whenever there was any occasion where liquor was served, or could be sneaked.

"Why did I do it?" she said. "To have fun, which I did have—or thought I did at the time. I was not as good-looking as my older sister and I often felt ill at ease and inadequate. But not when I drank. I could look in the mirror after a couple of glasses of wine and feel certain that I actually looked better."

Lana was clever enough so that she was able to disguise her drinking habits, including periods when she had to remain away from home because of acute hangovers, unaccounted-for scratches and bruises, and other painfully obvious evidence of bouts with the bottle. She completely lost her inhibitions and developed an increasingly lurid reputation. "I liked booze and sex at first," she admitted, "but then I completely lost control. I'd meet boys I had never seen before and hop into bed with them in a matter of hours, with no more hesitation than if they had asked me to dance. I'd wake up looking at a completely strange face, not knowing where I was or what had gone on."

Several times she was picked up by the police and jailed

overnight. Once she hit a girl friend over the head with a bar stool, gave her a concussion, and was charged with assault. She spent time in a number of urban detoxification centers and several "drying-out" camps in the country. She was treated for a variety of alcohol-related physical disorders, including malnutrition, jaundice, DTs, pancreatitis, and various withdrawal symptoms. She flunked out of school, lost most of her friends, and was considered pretty close to "hopeless."

Yet she was just beyond her eighteenth birthday.

Today, at twenty, she is recovered, a freshman at college, a volunteer peer counselor in an alcohol education program, and perhaps more solidly on her feet than a good many other youngsters who never faced the traumatic experiences she has undergone.

"Heretofore little had been known about teenage drinking habits or what causes a teenager to become an alcoholic," states a provocative book, *Twelve Young Women,** based on interviews with subjects whose drinking problems had started in their teens, along with a host of other problems, many of them alcohol-related.

"One thing is obvious from their stories," says the Introduction. "Each of the twelve young women drank heavily. The following statements indicate their drinking habits:

I loved it. I drank a lot. I drank to be drunk.

I could drink the boys under the table.

I drank down shots of tequila until I could hardly stand. Cool people drank all the time.

I always wanted to get out of it.

I would still be drinking after all had passed out.

"For most of the twelve young women, age thirteen seemed to be the turning point. This was when everything seemed to come together, including sex, grades, relationships, drinking, and other drug use."

The authors, Norm and Alexandra Southerby, report that

---

* See Appendix: Books, for how to order.

the girls all shared the feeling of not belonging, feeling apart from and out of touch with others. *Communication* was the vital link to normalcy that seemed to be missing.

"Throughout the lives of these women it is apparent that communication was lacking. They were, for whatever reasons, unable to communicate with their parents, teachers, friends, and, most importantly, with themselves."

Almost without exception, the subjects reported to the Southerbys that when they were in their teens and getting into trouble with booze, drugs, sex, studies, or a combination thereof, there were major communications gaps. The mother was "dull" or a "doormat" or taking her own escape route from life. The father was uncommunicative, away from home much of the time, or nonexistent. Many of the girls did not relate at all to their peers because of real or imagined inadequacies. They were constantly in conflict with their teachers, and unable to carry on any kind of meaningful dialogues with adults—even with ministers, priests, or counselors.

When the twelve finally began the long, painful turnaround that led back to a more normal existence, they did so because they were able to establish lines of communication with people who counted, who were interested, and who were in positions where they could help.

How do teenage drinkers feel about their plight?

The feelings of many teenagers in trouble with booze is summed up in this letter I received from "Jody," who prefers to remain anonymous:

Dear Mr. Cross:
I noticed in a newsletter. published by the NIAAA that you are writing a book on *Kids and Booze*. I am not much of an authority, since I am only seventeen, but I am a *kid* and I know a great deal—more than I wish I did—about *booze*. But maybe I can contribute a thought that you could pass along to parents, that is, if you can get what I'm saying and write it up more clearly than I'm able to. It's parents and teachers and other grown-ups who should realize this, so that perhaps some of them will do something about it when the opportunity arises.

Young people all over the country get into trouble because they drink too much, or when they are too young. I do not know anything about head counts, but people who do seem to know say that the proportions of those in trouble versus those who are not vary quite a bit from one location to another, but that there are few communities without some problems. When kids get into trouble *they usually do it with other kids.* Very few—at least around where I live—get into trouble all by themselves, except maybe those who are recluses and kind of mentally unbalanced.

I got into trouble with wine. A girl friend of mine had a serious problem with beer at parties and was frequently getting smashed and hauled home by a couple of boys and sneaked in through the cellar. But what happened? As soon as we (or most young people) get into a jam, we're yanked out of society, our society, and put into a kind of "solitary confinement." Adults somehow think that since we were getting messed up in a group we're going to get straightened out like a goal post if forced to face the misery by ourselves.

Well, it ain't necessarily so, as somebody's old song goes. I got nowhere in solitary. My parents tried everything—taking away all privileges, threats, sending me to a shrink (who needed help more than I did!), pleas, promises of rewards. Nothing got through. I wasn't ready. Then my father was transferred by his firm and we moved to a completely different community. Thank God! The county had a broad alcohol prevention and recovery program. I was right back in a group situation, but this time with kids *who wanted to help each other* beat the odds. They had all had it with booze, or drugs—some with both. Not one of them had to hack it alone, the way I had been forced to do.

Did it work? Now I'm an officer in my class, on the basketball team, and very active in our alcohol program. The most important thing is that *I don't drink*, and I can refuse drinks or alcoholic involvement without feeling self-conscious, put upon, or left out.

So please tell teachers, tell parents, tell all adults who have anything to do with what goes on in their community that this is the kind of program we really need: one that gets everyone involved, that brings the subject out into the open, that treats alcohol and alcohol abuse as something every person, every neighbor should be able to discuss.

If your town was being demoralized and the inhabitants sickened by air pollution, you wouldn't get far by having each citizen or family trying to counteract it independently, in secret. You'd have meetings, enlist the aid of many people, hold discussions, and take action. Well, what is problem drinking but another form of pollution —*body pollution?*

As we say in our meetings, thanks for listening,

Sincerely,
Jody

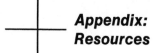

Appendix:
Resources

Where to get information and help

Immediate aid

If the situation is unbearable and you need instant counsel and relief, the best help may be as near as your telephone. Look up any of the following entries in your local telephone book or ask for directory assistance:

A.A. or Alcoholics Anonymous
Al-Anon
Alcoholism Consultation and Information Center
Alcoholism Services
National Council on Alcoholism

You may also find listings for state agencies. Look up your state, alphabetically, where you will find listings for departments and agencies. The proper organization will be found under "Alcohol," "Alcoholism," or "Drug Dependence."

Medical associations, hospitals, family consultation services, and the police can usually put you in contact with an individual or agency able to advise you.

Long-range information and counsel

Except in emergencies, your best approach is to look at the problem as one that has taken a long time developing and will require considerable time and application to solve. The following organizations can be helpful. Since they deal with thousands of cases and problems in a wide variety of situations, they need specific—

though brief—details, such as: the age, sex, and family status of the person involved; the kind of help you are seeking; current, or recent, situations that have been causing problems; any corrective or restorative action that has been taken or is in progress.

You can rest assured that these organizations will keep the matter *confidential*.

Al-Anon Family Group Headquarters
P.O. Box 182
Madison Square Station
New York, NY 10010
(212) 475-6110

Alcohol and Drug Problems Association
1101 15th Street, NW
Washington, DC 20005
(202) 452-0990

Alcoholics Anonymous World Services
Box 459
Grand Central Station
New York, NY 10017
(212) 686-1100

American Council on Alcohol Problems
119 Constitution Avenue, NE
Washington, DC 20002
(202) 543-2441

American Medical Association
535 North Dearborn Street
Chicago, IL 60610
(312) 751-6000

Blue Shield Association
211 East Chicago Avenue
Chicago, IL 60611
(312) 440-5500

Department of Health, Education and Welfare
National Institute on Alcohol Abuse and Alcoholism
P.O. Box 2345
Rockville, MD 20852
(301) 948-4450

National Council on Alcoholism
733 Third Avenue
New York, NY 10017
(212) 986-4433

Rutgers University
Center of Alcohol Studies
New Brunswick, NJ 08903
(201) 932-2190

Salvation Army
120 West 14th Street
New York, NY 10011
(212) 620-4900

Veterans Administration
Alcohol and Drug Dependent Service
810 Vermont Avenue, NW
Washington, DC 20420
(202) 389-5193

Further reading

Books

Addeo, Edmund G. and Jovita R. *Why Our Children Drink*. Englewood Cliffs, NJ: Prentice-Hall, 1975, 240 pages, out of print, $7.95. Why young people start to drink, why they continue, and why some abstain and others have problems.

Al-Anon Family Group Headquarters. *Al-Anon Faces Alcoholism*. New York: Al-Anon, P.O. Box 182, Madison Square Station, New York, NY 10010, 1975, 285 pages, $5.75. For everyone concerned with drinking problems; contains a section by outstanding professionals, a history of the organization, and an evaluation of its principles.

————. *Living with an Alcoholic*. New York: Al-Anon, 1978, 176 pages, $4.75. The history and purpose of Al-Anon and how it works, with real-life stories by parents, spouses, and children of alcoholics.

Alcoholics Anonymous. *Alcoholics Anonymous: The Story of How Many Thousands of Men and Women Have Recovered from Alcoholism*. New York: Alcoholics Anonymous, 1955, 578 pages, $5.95. The authorized A.A. reference and guide, describing the principles of the program and providing personal case histories of recovered alcoholics, old and young.

Ayars, Albert L., and Milgram, Gail G. *The Teenager and Alcohol.* New York: Richards Rosen Press, 1970, 96 pages, $7.97. Short, informative, recommended by the National Institute of Alcohol Abuse and Alcoholism.

Bacon, Margaret, and Jones, M. B. *Teenage Drinking.* New York: Thomas Y. Crowell, 1971, 228 pages, $6.95. A reliable reference on attitudes about drinking, peer pressures, how to understand problems that arise, and where to obtain help.

Englebardt, Stanley L. *Kids and Alcohol—the Deadliest Drug.* New York: Lothrop, Lee and Shepard Co., 1975, 64 pages, $4.50. Uses the scare approach, but can be useful.

Fleming, Alice. *Alcohol: The Delightful Poison.* New York: Delacorte Press, 1976, 138 pages, $6.95. A history of alcohol in the life of man for young readers, ten and up; one chapter discusses the medical effects of alcohol on young people.

Haskins, James. *Teen-age Alcholism.* New York: Hawthorn Books, 1976, 136 pages, hardcover $6.95, paperback $2.95. Provides examples of alcoholism, what it is, and why and how teenagers drink.

Jordan, Donald K. *Alcohol Abuse Prevention: A Comprehensive Guide for Youth Organizations.* Boys' Club of America Project TEAM, 1978.

Lee, Essie E. *Alcohol—Proof of What?* New York: Julian Messner, 1976, 91 pages, $6.25. Written for adolescents, based on the author's research into the drinking habits and outlook of high school students.

————, and Israel, Elaine. *Alcohol and You.* New York: Julian Messner, 1975, 64 pages, $6.25. Written for youth, a helpful look at the attitudes of young people toward drinking.

Milgram, Gail G. *What Is Alcohol? And Why Do People Drink?* Center of Alcohol Studies, Rutgers University, 1975, 25 pages, 75¢. Packed with information, diagrams, and illustrations; the author, a knowledgable authority, writes with clarity and insight.

Silverstein, Alvin and Virginia B. *Alcoholism.* Philadelphia: J. B. Lippincott Company, 1975, 128 pages, $5.50. Presents the facts on alcohol use and abuse and is helpful for making decisions about drinking.

Southerby, Norm and Alexandra. *Twelve Young Women.* Southerby and Associates, P.O. Box 15403, Long Beach, CA 90815, 1975, 158 pages, $4.95. A fascinating account of the lives of twelve young women whose personalities, problems, and circumstances led them into alcoholism.

Wagner, Robin S. *Sarah T: Portrait of a Teen-age Alcoholic.* New York: Ballantine Books, 1976, 120 pages, paperback, $1.50. This account, based on real life, looks at what it is like to be young and an alcoholic.

Pamphlets

Al-Anon Family Group Headquarters. *Alcoholism the Family Disease* (25¢). *A Guide for the Family of the Alcoholic* (10¢). *So You Love an Alcoholic* (5¢). These and other small publications are usually available at no cost from local offices of Al-Anon.

Alcoholic Anonymous. Dozens of small publications are available at no cost on A.A. programs, several of which are focused specifically on youthful drinkers, from Alcoholics Anonymous World Services, Inc., Box 459, Grand Central Station, New York, NY 10016, or from any local A.A. group.

DISCUS. *No One Answer: A Closer Look at Teenage Drinking* (free). *If You Choose to Drink, Drink Responsibly* (free). DISCUS, Suite 1300, 425 13th Street, NW, Washington, DC 20004.

National Clearinghouse for Alcohol Information. Many publications are available at no cost by writing: National Clearinghouse for Alcohol Information, P.O. Box 2345, Rockville, MD 20852. Examples: Kit, "Package on Youth," includes pamphlets, reprints, and posters; *Alcohol: A Family Affair* (a PTA pamphlet).

National Council on Alcoholism. *Alcohol: Pleasures and Problems* (45¢). *Alcohol: The New Teen-age Turn-On* ($1.25). *Alcohol and the Adolescent* (free). *Alcoholic Beverages: Social Use—or Sick Abuse?* (25¢). These and other publications (many at no cost) available from Publications Department, National Council on Alcoholism, 733 Third Avenue, New York, NY 10017.

Also available is a "Blood Alcohol Content Wheel" (35¢), which shows how much alcohol gets into the blood according to such factors as number of ounces imbibed, time involved, and weight of the drinker.

Public Affairs Pamphlets. *The New Alcoholics: Teen-agers,* #499 (free). *How to Help the Alcoholic,* #452 (free). *Alcoholism—A Sick-*

ness That Can Be Beaten, #118A (50¢). Other small publications as well as the above can be obtained by writing Public Affairs Pamphlets, 381 Park Avenue South, New York, NY 10016.

Rutgers. *How Alcohol Affects the Body,* Mark Keller (25¢). *What the Body Does with Alcohol,* Leon A. Greenberg (25¢). *What Shall We Teach the Young about Drinking?* Robert D. Russell (25¢). *Teen-age Drinking, Drug Use, and Social Correlates,* Henry Wechsler and Denise Thum (30¢). These and many other books and pamphlets can be obtained from Rutgers Center of Alcohol Studies, Rutgers University, New Brunswick, NJ 08903.

U.S. Department of Transportation. *How to Talk to Your Teenager About Drinking and Driving* (free). *How to Keep the Life of the Party Alive* (free). Write U.S. Department of Transportation, National Highway Traffic Safety Administration, Washington, DC 20590.

U.S. Government Printing Office. *Thinking About Drinking,* #1683 (50¢). *Drinking Etiquette: For Those Who Drink and Those Who Don't,* DHEW Publication No. (ADM) 77-305 (40¢). *Alcohol: Some Questions and Answers,* #HSM 71-9048 (35¢). *The Drinking Question—Honest Answers to Questions Teen-agers Ask About Drinking,* #017-024-00473-1 (55¢). Order from: Superintendent of Documents, U.S. Government Printing Office, Washington, DC 20402.

U.S. Jaycees. *Drinking Myths* (free). A 24-page illustrated pamphlet that dissolves some of the falsehoods and fallacies about drinking. U.S. Jaycees, Box 7, Tulsa, OK 74102.

———— *Understanding How We Teach and Influence Children About Alcohol* ($1.00). A very useful 52-page pocket book that discusses alcohol from the viewpoints of both parents and children. With illustrations, check lists, and Q&A sections. U.S. Jaycees, Box 7, Tulsa, OK 74102.

Index